MAK

T0165069

PRE-MED
COUNT

EVERYTHING I WISH
I'D KNOWN BEFORE
APPLYING *(Successfully)*
TO MEDICAL SCHOOL

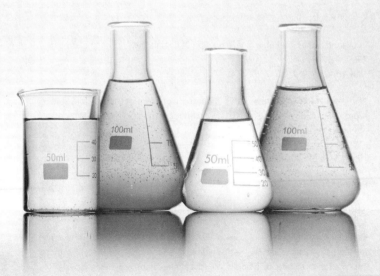

ELISABETH FASSAS, B.S., MSc.

© 2020 Kaplan, Inc.

Published by Kaplan Publishing, a division of Kaplan, Inc.
750 Third Avenue
New York, NY 10017

10 9 8 7 6 5 4 3 2 1

Printed in Canada

ISBN: 978-1-5062-5818-8

Kaplan Publishing print books are available at special quantity discounts to use for sales promotions, employee premiums, or educational purposes. For more information or to purchase books, please call the Simon & Schuster special sales department at 866-506-1949.

Acknowledgements

To A, V, A, and C—thank you for all of your love and support consistently.

To the Notes and Ranvier and the friends and peers who talked me through their admissions process and offered words of wisdom, thank you for your time and your openness.

Table of Contents

INTRODUCTION

So you want to go to medical school, huh? Fantastic!

I'm sure you are equal parts excited and stressed about this plan—or at least, I'm sure there will be times over the next few years when you will be.

Your four years (or more) of pre-med will be riddled with decisions and wrought with opportunity for stress, anxiety, and comparison to others. It will also set you up to get successfully into and through medical school, where you will be privileged enough to gain the knowledge necessary to serve your patients and your community in a way only doctors can.

It's going to be amazing! And you have picked up a great resource to help you through this process. This book is a compilation of everything you need to know about and think about as you apply to medical school, complete with insiders' tips, tricks, and knowledge, and pep talks from pre-med advisors, admissions officers, and students who are either going through or have just finished this process.

My name is Elisabeth and I am the narrator of this story. I have successfully made it to other side, having received my coveted acceptance to medical school, and want to use my 20/20 hindsight to shine some light on some common pitfalls. I probably won't help you avoid them all, but maybe I can help with a few as you traverse the long and winding road to a medical school admission.

Let's talk about that road for a second. Most available resources, your pre-professional advisors, and everyone who has made it to the finish line presents it, in my experience, as a single-lane street. You pass academics, extracurricular activities, research, and clinical experience and then BOOM, you land yourself in a matriculating class. At least, that's how I had visualized it before getting started.

What most pre-meds will tell you, however, is that this road is riddled with potholes, dead ends, and intersections that will require you to choose to turn one way or the other. Your ability to trek through to the end depends on making millions of decisions that all seem, in their own right, infinitely impactful. Chances are, you will spend many, *many* days of your pre-med years feeling like you're running through quicksand. Every choice you make will necessarily eliminate the possibility for another, and you will undoubtedly second-guess yourself. It is unavoidable: the medical school application process is just transparent enough to make you feel like everyone around you is doing something more interesting than you are, and just opaque enough to make you feel as though you've spent the last four years playing Russian roulette blindfolded.

I, and (as I found out later) many of my friends and peers, spent a long time obsessing over all of the things we *could have* done, all of the tick boxes we *could have* checked, and the experience points we *could have* collected. If you take nothing else from this book, this is the most important lesson: as you look backward to the path you didn't take, you will miss the potholes ahead of you and move more slowly than if you had forged ahead with your full might and attention. Oh, and that whatever you do is probably much more interesting when you put it on paper than you thought it would be when you were doing it.

I began to write this resource because I realized a very sobering fact about the medical school application process and the academic environments within which students' stories are playing out every day. Universities, even those with plenty of resources and staff, often fall short in the number of pre-professional advisors they have available for students to access. Now, the ones they do have (at least the ones I know), are absolute superheroes. They field emails from anxious students and help to create action plans and strategies that help their students get into their dream schools. The problem is that there are often too few advisors to go around when students are in college. An even bigger problem is that after graduation, those resources all but disappear for alumni, leaving students who decide to pursue medicine relatively late in the game, or otherwise nontraditional students, with the short end of the stick in terms of solid, industry-informed advice about the nuances of the application process. This is problematic because even for the perfect applicant the average acceptance rate still hovers at around 7% per medical school, and honestly, I think we each need all the help we can get.

I wrote this book fresh out of the medical school application process, after spending nearly an entire year maneuvering through what felt like a minefield. I had to make thousands of little decisions about the different pieces of my application without really knowing the criteria that my choices would be judged against. So, I set out to answer the million-dollar question: What are medical school admissions committees looking for anyway?

If you are a current student, I hope this book will provide guidance and direction as you plan out your personal journey to medical school. If you are finished with your pre-med years and are looking to apply, I hope this book will help frame the experiences you have amassed in the best possible light.

To do this, I spent the last several months on a quest to pick the brains of as many current and former pre-meds, admissions officers, and pre-med advisors as possible, to determine what applicants can do to be most successful in this process. The quotes herein are from real people offering real advice, but the student scenarios they describe are indicative of *types* of students, rather than actual students.

For all applicants, aspiring applicants, and cheer squads to a very special pre-med, this book can serve three main purposes:

1. To help you organize your pre-med-related thoughts in a way that will keep you focused on the core of

your value add, without going bonkers over all the conflicting advice out there;

2. To teach you to get into the heads of the admissions committees that will be considering your candidacy, so you can test your brilliant ideas as you design your journey to medicine; and

3. To remind you that you are not the only one confused and anxious about this process, no matter how often it may seem like it.

Before we dive in, I want to give you some calming words that you can come back to throughout this process when you need some perspective:

No one who really wanted to be a doctor didn't get there eventually.

The acceptance rate to medical school throughout the country has hovered around 40% for the past three years. This means that many applicants were not necessarily accepted their first time around. With some appropriate application tweaks, however, everyone has the potential to get there at some point.

This is not meant to stress you out. Honestly, if you are reading this book, you are already thinking about how to craft your application, so you are probably already ahead of the game. All I am trying to say with that admittedly terrifying statistic is that your worst-case scenario has you simply delaying acceptance for a year. Your life is not over, and you *will* eventually become a doctor.

A delay. That is all.

Let that sink in for a second, and let it offer you some perspective during the late nights where anxieties about the future may keep you up.

Everyone is struggling.

I know, I know. Suzie got an A on her biochemistry exam and told you she didn't study at all. Organic chemistry looks like a bunch of odd shapes and you are the *only* one in the *whole* class who isn't getting it.

I know it must seem that way. But take it from someone who was always too proud to admit when something was hard and too ashamed to divulge a poor test grade: most people are fantastic at acting cool when they are really struggling just as much as you. I promise you are not alone, as much as it may seem like it.

The day-to-day challenges that you face will provide you with the fodder you need to write a convincing story on your application.

I was told in my very first medical school interview, where I sheepishly admitted being incredibly nervous and knowing that my grades did not meet the average for admitted students at this particular university, that "interesting paths make for fantastic medical students." At the time I was too stressed during this interview to clarify, but what I have taken it to mean as I've moved away from this entire process is that the challenges that you will face in the time leading up to your application will inevitably lead to a compelling application that the human on the other end of the screen will enjoy reading and relate to. Try to feel grateful when they do arise and keep looking for the lessons hidden under the mess.

You don't have to cure cancer to get into medical school.

In fact, no one who ever went to medical school has. I know it will seem like everyone around you is making fantastic strides in their research and community service activities and that your pursuits seem insignificant in comparison. I also know that you're excited to become a neurosurgeon right now and can't possibly wait any longer. You won't get there overnight though, and no one is expecting you to, so take a breath and try to enjoy this pre-med ride.

Just for reading this compilation of advice and personal anecdotes, you will undoubtedly be better off than I was. You will hopefully look back and question yourself less often and commit with greater certainty to the choices you make when building your application. You will have the confidence to convince yourself, your parents, your advisors, and, ultimately, your admissions committees of the reasons behind your choices and why they will help shape you into an incredible doctor. I'm so excited you have elected to take me on this journey with you!

Let's get started.

APPLICATION TIMELINE

JUNE

T minus 15 months to matriculation, you should be ready to submit your primary application and the associated fees. The primary application, which you will submit directly to American Medical College Application Service (AMCAS), will include the following pieces:

- Demographics, parental, and personal information

- Academic record (the information contained in your transcript)

- MCAT (Medical College Admission Test) scores (You don't necessarily need these at the time you submit your primary, but must at least be able to say when you plan on testing. This topic will be covered later.)

- Activities list

- Personal statement

- Letters of recommendation

- List of schools to which you are applying

July

Secondary application invitations will start coming in from (almost) all of your schools. You will likely be writing these applications well into August.

September–January

Interview season for most schools. Some may also extend their interview seasons into August or February, depending on the size of their incoming class.

September–March

Schools will begin sending out positive, negative, or "we're not sure yet" responses to candidates who have interviewed. Yes, because each school gets to determine its own timing, it is very possible that you may have interviewed at one school and have received a definitive answer on the state of your candidacy there without even knowing if you've been invited for an interview at others.

April 30

The last day that candidates are allowed to hold multiple acceptances to medical school. After this date, candidates are required to commit to one school via AMCAS and to withdraw their applications from any other school to which they hold an acceptance. You are permitted, however, to hold an application on a waitlist at another school after this date.

May 1

You are most likely to hear back from schools that have waitlisted you at this point, and into the early summer as schools will be working to fill spots previously held by students with multiple acceptances.

DESIGNING YOUR PRE-MED YEARS | 2

The pre-medical years, including the required classes and the application process, have been carefully designed to filter out the students not fully committed or not experienced enough…Unfortunately, they also create a fair bit of pain and suffering for everyone else.

PRE-MED YEARS— THE PARADOX

Your college years are meant to be the best years of your life. They are often referred to as "formative," where you'll find yourself, or create yourself, or something like that. You will learn how to become independent, make ramen noodles taste edible, go out until 3 AM, and show up at your 8 AM lecture without missing a beat, hangover free and green smoothie in tow. These are truly the golden years. It is a unique time when you and your friends will make questionable choices that result in fond memories.

Now all of that may be true, especially if you live on a college campus, and more so if you don't have a medical school application looming over your head. It will feel to you that your non-pre-med friends and peers will lead lives of fun adventures and late nights. There will be plenty of people living their college experience to the fullest, with all of the parties, *a cappella* concerts, football games, and dormwide sleepovers that entails. Actually, if you take a second to imagine your version of *the* college experience, I can guarantee someone you know will be living it, and I can (almost) guarantee that someone won't be you. If you are really intent on going to medical school, your grades and extracurriculars will almost always take precedence over "the college experience," and that will inevitably cause friction and annoyance in your life.

This is where the struggle of the pre-med student begins. Your college years are meant to be a time for you to explore your interests, develop a hobby, grow into a well-rounded person, build lasting relationships with your peers, and discover your passions. You know, all the stuff they write in the brochures and put in the movies. The undergraduate experience is the gem of the American education system— the space for this type of personal development at an ideal time in your life is a truly unique opportunity.

In addition to all of that self-exploration, though, medical school aspirants must also prove their ability to take on the medical school curriculum in a variety of ways. They need to develop interview skills, immerse themselves in the field of medicine, and get stellar grades, all the while convincing themselves (and future admissions officers) that they actually want to go into medicine in the first place.

And, as if all of that didn't keep you busy enough already, you also have to fit in time to eat, sleep, study, have a social life, remain an active participant in your family, and find a way to pay for it all! If that seems like a lot, don't worry, you're not crazy (because it absolutely is). And you're not alone in feeling that way. If you've taken a stab at doing it all at once, become overwhelmed, and thought about reassessing your career choice, well, you're not the only one.

I remember the first time in my college career I tried to talk myself out of becoming a doctor. It was Halloween of freshman year (yeah, I know, it seems like the doubts crept in pretty early for me), and *everyone* I knew was going out. I couldn't even count the number of parties that were happening, but I did know that I was missing every single one of them because my Calculus II professor thought that Friday, November 1 (at 9 AM, mind you), would be a great day to schedule our midterm.

Womp.

Now, you may or may not know that Chipotle has $2 burritos on Halloween if you show up in costume. Having suffered through an entire day of calculus practice problems and the unbearable weight of my FOMO (fear of missing out) as my four suitemates dressed up as M&M's and hit the town, I was determined to *at least* not miss the greatest Chipotle day of the year. However, I did not have any time to waste cobbling a costume together.

To make a long story short, I walked into Chipotle with a messy bun and no makeup, wearing pajamas (and, if memory serves, a horrific neon yellow shirt because *HELLOOO* I have a Calc II midterm this week and want to go to medical school so who has time for laundry?) and had a very lively discussion with the man wrapping my burrito about whether or not "college student with an exam tomorrow" counts as a costume—a true low point in my college career, I remember thinking. Ha! Little did I know what was still to come.

See? I told you you're not alone!

The problem for those of you who have decided that medicine is the path for you—and for those of you still on the fence about it—is that these precious, formative, incredibly fun years also happen to overlap with the years in which you must prove your potential to become a doctor. In order to enjoy yourself while putting your best foot forward when submitting your medical school application, these years have to be productive but social, focused but exploratory, successful but challenging. It is in these dichotomies that many pre-med students get lost.

The good news is that thousands of people have navigated this path before, and you can too.

So now that I have thoroughly stressed you out and hopefully given you something to look forward to, let's dive into this crazy mess of a journey!

Compete with Yourself, Not Others

Picture this: You meet for the first time a group of aspiring pre-meds (I'm sure it didn't take long, we tend to be a fairly vocal tribe). You are all chatting about your plans, medicine, shadowing opportunities, and all is well. You feel one with the pack, a part of this giant pre-med, we-don't-really-know-what-we're-doing-but-are-super-excited-to-be-here family, and it's thrilling and exciting and feels so close that you can almost smell the formaldehyde.

Then someone starts talking about their childhood illness or their sick parent, and the doctors who helped them through that experience. They speak about hospitals and medication regimens with an intimacy that is foreign to you and you find yourself thinking, *Damn! I wish I had a story like that!*

I know. It sounds like this girl has her personal statement already written and that you are already behind the curve by not having this compelling personal experience that can help explain why you began your journey to physicianship.

Do not be alarmed.

Yes, you did just get annoyed that you have never experienced a horrible illness and that your family members are alive and well. I'll bet you just attempted to dramatize your less serious life experiences to keep up with these "I-want-to-be-a-doctor-and-I-know-why" folks.

If this isn't the case, then 1) congratulations, you are likely a much more chilled-out human being than I am, and 2) have no fear, my friend, as your time will definitely come.

Either way, no worries. I guarantee you will have plenty of time to get at the core of exactly why you want to be a doctor in a way that is unique to you.

Setting Yourself Up for Success

It's Tuesday, November 2. The Halloweekend craze is over, and you feel overwhelmed by the amount of work you have to do.

The process of stressing yourself out so you feel like you aren't able to accomplish anything (or everything gets half done) and the subsequent spiral that leads to the inevitable "I-won't-get-into-med-school-if-I-don't… [fill in the blank] panic can be whittled down to five steps. The process is both so simple and so predictable that if you walk across a college campus and watch students as they race from class to activity to library, you can practically see it unfolding on their faces.

Stage 1: Overbooking Yourself

It's early November. Thanksgiving is in sight, but not close enough to provide any real peace. It is a stressful time in the semester. The work keeps piling on with final projects and midterm exams, and you regret all those nights at the beginning of the semester when you were just a *little* less productive. Not to mention, everyone you know is out apple picking and stomping through leaves to get the perfect #insta while you spend the "best years of your life" in the library.

You now have exactly two days to study for your organic chemistry midterm exam *and* read 150 pages for your anthropology class *and* write up a lab report for organic chemistry lab (because of course they would schedule those to be due in the same week).

That yoga class you promised to go to is scheduled for 7:30 PM tonight. Sleep is usually the first thing to go, because pulling all-nighters is what all college kids do, right?

Then cooking and eating nutritious meals is next; how good do those vending machine chips look when you haven't had time to go grocery shopping in two weeks and all you have in your fridge are a jar of old mustard and a wilting head of lettuce?

Next come social outings of any kind. Sorry Lizzie, no time to celebrate your birthday this week—some of us are trying to get into medical school, okay?

Now you are fatigued, a little miserable, and bitterly scrolling through your social media feeds looking at all the fun everyone else is having. But you can't seem to pay attention in any of your lectures and are spending like, I don't know, $12 a day on iced coffee. And yet, even after all these sacrifices, you are still behind.

Before you know it, you've spent 45 minutes strategically laying out a plan to fulfill four days' worth of work and activities in two.

STAGE 2: THE REVENGE OF THE IGNORED

During this period, all those corners you cut and sleep you lost start to catch up with you. You are behind and stressed, and there is no free time for you to catch your breath! And so the negotiations begin…

You cut out everything nonacademic that you can, but now things are getting super serious. You begin to skimp on some of your lower-intensity classes. "Okay," you reason. "Maybe I don't have to read all 150 pages of this English literature book. I mean, I just have to get the gist, right? As long as I scan scrape up some intelligent-sounding comment in the discussion section it should be fine."

And then come the calculations…

"If I get all of the attendance points for organic chemistry and commit to studying really hard for the final, then maybe I can get away with a B on the exam and still get an A- in the class. Plus, everyone I've talked to seems to be as unprepared as I am for this exam, so as long as I'm at the curve that should be fine… Now, how many hours of studying orgo will get me a B…?"

Stage 3: Acceptance

This is when you start debating with yourself about what you can permanently go without.

"You know what? I'll just stop studying for my Spanish class again. I mean, it's not like it's physics, right? Oh, and no more yoga! Who needs all that breathing, anyway?"

STAGE 4: PANIC

This is the point at which it really becomes visible to you and to your loved ones that you actually are deeply, *deeply* stressed, which might have implications for your mental health now and down the road. You worry that some things are just too important to cut out of your life completely. I mean, you signed up to be a volunteer translator at the women's shelter for a reason, right? You are a good, kind person who likes to do good in the world, but also probably because you thought this kind of thing would fill a gap in your application, the gap that you've convinced yourself is there. Plus, you've already put so much time and effort into building a community at that center, and are sure you could write about it in beautiful prose that subtly highlights both your love of helping people and your ability to communicate in Spanish!

Before you know it, you realize that all the time you spent worrying about your schedule could've been used studying for that Spanish quiz. Not the best use of time, my friend.

STAGE 5: ACCEPTANCE...AGAIN

You finally come to terms with the fact that it is not possible to squeeze eight hours of sleep, two hours of socializing, four hours of class, six hours of studying, three hours of volunteering, four hours of shadowing, one hour of exercise, and some spare minutes to inhale a sandwich all into a single day. You will also realize, if you haven't already, that despite your best intentions, you will not be the exception to this rule.

Here's an example of how this played out in my life. My first semester of sophomore year was particularly busy. That was on purpose, by the way. I typically work most productively under pressure and thought that it would be a *brilliant* move to willingly overbook myself. High-pressure semester = productive semester, no?

I'm sure you can predict where this little anecdote is going.

During one particularly busy week, I had a physics midterm on Tuesday and a biochemistry midterm on Thursday. Naturally, my hopes of getting caught up on my schoolwork during the semester had not panned out as I had hoped. I felt more comfortable with biochemistry than I did with physics, so I planned to focus all of my attention on physics until the exam, then start studying for biochemistry after that.

Now, please do not be fooled (as I was) into thinking that this was somehow a strategic choice. I actually deliberately planned to not give myself enough time to prepare for an exam in a subject in which I could have gotten an A. I'm not kidding. These were things that I, and many of my classmates, did because there simply is not enough space in that ol' noggin for both subjects at the same time— especially when you haven't slept a full night or eaten a vegetable in three months.

So what came of my brilliant plan? Not only did I perform poorly on my physics exam, but I also performed poorly on my biochemistry exam, a subject that I could have reasonably gotten an A in if I had dedicated enough focused time to studying.

So then what do you about all this? How do you meet the seemingly insurmountable goals of your ideal medical school when there are only 24 hours in a day and only so many all-nighters you can pull before you collapse from exhaustion?

If you're nodding your head as you read this, I'm not surprised. This process of running yourself into the ground via borrowing energy and focus from the next day and trying to tack it onto the current one doesn't work, even though almost everyone will insist on giving it the old college try.

Instead, here are some things that do work. Warning: I am not going to say anything super-groundbreaking in the paragraphs that follow, because the discovery you made— that it's not possible to do everything at the same time and still be well rested, happy, and productive—was 100% true. However, there are some things you can do to get a little more bang for your buck throughout your negotiations with yourself.

MAKE YOUR SCHEDULE WORK FOR YOU

Most U.S. universities are set up to give you maximum flexibility when designing your curriculum. Other than having to follow some guidelines for prerequisite classes and trying to fit in all of your required classes before taking the MCAT, there are few limitations on what you can do. You can design your schedule to maximize your chances of success. This freedom is spectacular—and wholly undervalued by most undergraduates!

What this means is that by making your own schedule, you can maximize your chances of graduating with a stellar GPA. Your professors are generally able to tell you when projects, papers, midterms, and final exams are due in advance. Spend an hour in the first week of your semester mapping out those dates to make sure there are no conflicts between the classes. Think about how much better I could have performed on my biochemistry exam if I didn't also have to take a physics exam that week.

A semester is usually only about 12 weeks long. By the time you get your schedules from your professors, you should know when and where your stress/work levels will peak. Do you work best with high-stress weeks sandwiched between weeks that are much more relaxed? Are you burned out by the last day of finals period? Use this information to your advantage: see if you can save one of those classes for a different semester, and don't take a class that has its final scheduled for that day. Whatever your ideal is, make it so. If at all possible, you should create a schedule that is achievable and maximizes your chances of success.

MAKE THAT FIRST WEEKEND YOUR SUCCESS STORY

I have a theory that I (unfortunately) managed to prove each of my eight semesters of college. The theory says that how productive you manage to be in the first weekend of the semester will determine if you will be behind or ahead of schedule. Think about it. That first weekend is the only time you have "free," before extracurriculars kick into high gear and when you aren't yet expected to really know anything.

You have this golden opportunity of two *whole* days to get ahead of the curve, give yourself a cushion, and prepare for the barrage of reading and PowerPoint slides that lie ahead. However, almost no one does it (or at least, that's what I told myself). Before you know it, it's Monday morning and everything is in full swing again. The summer, or winter break, or weekend that just passed is nothing but a faint, joyful memory, and you have 12 chapters of *Jane Eyre* to read, two problem sets to solve, and 150 flashcards to memorize.

That first weekend of your semester, when everything seems blissful and happy and like things aren't going to be so bad after all, can be a missed opportunity if you're not careful. Take those extra couple "light" days at the start of each semester as an opportunity to start off on the right foot— not as an extra two days of summer vacation/winter break/ weekend. Your grades, mental health, and sanity will all thank you later.

PROTECT YOUR NONNEGOTIABLES

Pick one thing that is absolutely nonnegotiable for you in your day. Is it an hour-long workout, an hour of your favorite sitcom to help you wind down at the end of the day, or time to cook and eat something healthy? Whatever that one thing is that makes you a healthy, functional, and happy human being is the one thing you need to carve out time for. I guarantee that the marginal gain achieved from one extra hour of studying (or stressing about studying) won't benefit you in the long run as much as that nonnegotiable window of "you time."

MAKE A SCHEDULE AND STICK TO IT

Groundbreaking advice, right? However, it is harder to implement than to say, but it's undoubtedly worth the effort.

DESIGN A SCHEDULE YOU ACTUALLY LIKE

Commit to doing tasks you actually enjoy instead of what you think will sound appealing to an admissions committee. Spoiler: they don't really care what you do, just how you do it.

For example, throughout my undergraduate career I spent two years working in a research lab. However, I was not really committed to the work and it showed. Although I learned a lot (including the fact that lab work was not where my career was headed, medical or otherwise), the experience was not meaningful to me because I never invested in it. When it came time to write about it, I found myself struggling to come up with the seven hundred characters that each activity gets in the description section of the application. I remember being upset with myself. I had spent too much time in this environment to omit it from my application, but felt I had wasted an opportunity to speak passionately about something I had enjoyed (not to mention all the time spent doing the work)—all because I was *sure* that I *had* to pursue lab-based research in order to get into medical school!

What ended up happening was that I shifted away from what I thought the admissions committee would want to read and into a topic that I could actually speak about compellingly. I realized, after two years of lab work and months of slaving over secondary applications, that the doctor I aspired to be was not one who would simultaneously be running a lab and making pharmaceutical discoveries for drug trials. So then, what did I value in a doctor? How did I see myself serving my patients, and what groups of patients was I setting myself up to serve?

I answered these questions in my junior year of college, when I found myself very happily involved in a sociological research project outside the lab. This project looked at levels of poverty in my hometown and assessed how poverty influenced the ways people interacted with the medical profession, via their family doctors and local hospitals. It turns out I was passionate about research—just not about the type I had originally been working on in the lab.

Nevertheless, I tried to keep a leg in both doors for almost an *entire year.* That is how long it took me to come to terms with the fact that I would not be entering the application cycle with a publication in a prestigious scientific journal. Coming to this conclusion was far from easy, as I mourned my perceived inability to contribute to my chosen career field and questioned whether or not medicine was even the right path for me. After all, the research I was aligning myself with and truly enjoying was sociological research. It took me months to reconcile what I had convinced myself were two different passions: medicine, and the ways peoples' environments affect their interaction with their healthcare system.

I was sure that I had made the wrong decision from the beginning. Actually, everything seemed wrong. By my junior year, my peers who had properly committed to the lab they had been with since freshman year were publishing papers and engaging in conversations with professors and grant committees about their projects. I was struggling to get networked in a completely new field—one that I was not majoring in (it was too late to switch and still graduate on time) and had very little to show for why I was driven to switch in the first place.

When I finally decided the theme of my application would be healthcare access and not the oncology research I had committed to in my first and second years, I had to give myself time to show commitment and personal growth on this new track. I basically forced myself into a gap year at precisely the time I should have been applying to medical school. The result: the highlight of my application was my project that looked at the ways people from different socioeconomic backgrounds interact with the healthcare profession and the impact this has on their health outcomes. I had committed many more hours to the lab-based research I didn't love. But it didn't matter—not on my application or in my interview. Because ultimately, it's not the hours you put in that matter, but what you do with them.

CRAFTING YOUR NARRATIVE

The medical school application is the culmination of all of your pre-med years, where you finally get to show an admissions committee how qualified, prepared, and excited you are to dive into medical school and begin becoming the doctor you have always dreamed of. It is an incredible process that can seem daunting until you open AMCAS and get cracking on it.

I'm going to attempt to demystify the medical school application in the following section.

The entire application is a few pages on AMCAS, where you will be asked to distill out the last four years of your life to 15 key experiences, along with a 5,300-character personal statement where you get to tell your whole "why medicine" story. You will get only seven hundred characters to write about each of the 15 activities (it might as well be a professional Twitter post), except for a few special ones, for which you will be granted the privilege of an extra 1,325 characters. This is not really enough space to explain any details of your story or what you think went wrong in your journey. No one will question decisions such as why you didn't pursue a lab experience your sophomore summer or why your choices are different than those of seemingly every other pre-med you have ever met.

The point is, after three or four years of building up an arsenal of experiences, you will only be given a tiny cabinet to fill. That means that you will have more than enough content to fill up your application. Don't worry about jumping on every opportunity that comes your way, and instead focus on pursuing what really interests and excites you. The worst thing you can do is have too many experiences to list, but none you can write about extensively. Remember that the people reading your applications have read millions just like yours and can differentiate real passion from feigned excitement.

The list of potential experiences is fairly minimal when you think about it. We are all doing the same things in different locations and talking about them in the same way with the same language. The important thing is not what you're doing, but *why* you are doing it. There are skills that a committee is looking for in every applicant, based on what a patient is looking for in their doctor. These skills may include:

- The commitment, respect, patience, and strength of character to take on the ultimate service job;

- The drive and passion to see through your education and training;

- The desire to be a lifelong learner and to serve your patients for decades to come; and

- The ability to empathize with a total stranger and to dedicate yourself wholly to their care.

These are traits inherent in most people who have adopted medicine as their calling. However, they need to be nurtured and refined, and, when the time comes, illustrated so the committee reading your application knows that you want this as much as you do. You are not 17 pages on the AMCAS, nor can you be distilled into 10,000 words. But you can bet that those words will represent the best pieces of you.

THE APPLICATION

Something I have observed about myself and my fellow pre-meds over the years is that we tend to be a pretty critical bunch. There is so much chatter about the perfect applicant: 4.0 GPA, 528 MCAT, has discovered a protein to cure Alzheimer's (which he will casually mention in a humble-brag Facebook post), saves puppies from burning buildings in his free time—you know the type. Now I'm sure this person is out there somewhere (and if it's you reading this, you can probably stop), but don't worry, he is *far* from the average applicant.

Here are some tips for preparing to submit an application:

1. Start framing what you do or what you have done as accomplishments rather than prerequisites.

2. The secret to becoming a successful applicant is not what you did, but *why* you did it and what you learned.

3. An admissions committee is trying to see on your application if you have what it takes to succeed in possibly the most grueling four years of your life (and I'm not talking about the pre-med years).

4. There is no cookie-cutter doctor.

Let's look at these closer.

START FRAMING

Just because "volunteer work" is on this elusive list of "things you have to do to get into med school," it does not mean that everyone is doing it and does not diminish the fact that you have done it. Focus on your "wins," and treat them as such.

THE WHY AND WHAT

You are not going to reinvent the wheel. Almost every applicant with a serious commitment and desire to become a medical student has some combination or variation of the following on their resume: volunteer work, research experience, clinical experience, and a solid academic record. I have no doubt that the project you are working on is super cool and interesting and different, but at the end of the day, it is just a project like all the interesting and different ones that all your fellow applicants are doing. So then what? The key is not to impress a committee with your responsibilities, title, or even institutional affiliation, but rather with your maturity and understanding of what medical school and your ultimate aspiration to a medical career actually entail. Which brings me to point #3.

The Admissions Committee

Your application must reflect the skills, temperament, and commitment I'm sure you have if you want to put yourself through the academic boot camp that is medical school. They want to know that you have the potential to become a good physician, and all they have to go on to determine how true that is are the 17 pages you will submit (plus maybe some secondary application materials). They are looking for grit, strength of character, emotional intelligence, and patience—as well as intellectual aptitude, glowing recommendations, and meaningful extracurricular activities. They are scanning your application for hints of what you can bring to your class across those dimensions.

Using the application to show how busy you are and how hard you've worked since starting college will dilute the work you have done. Everyone is busy, everyone has worked. Reminding a committee of that with the precious 5,300 characters you have in your personal statement will only waste words. Instead, use that space to color the image you are trying to convey.

A lot of this will come from the writing itself. For example, "I went into the lab early on a Saturday morning to call potential patients for a clinical trial I was working on" paints a very different picture about who you are and what drives you than, "The conversation I had with Patient X about the hope this drug offers her and her family was all I needed to power through an early Saturday morning session," while providing a committee the same information about the depth of your involvement in the project. One is trying to show that you are busy, while the other shows *what drives you* to be busy.

At the end of the day, you are all taking the same steps toward admission. A wealth of information is available through pre-professional advisors, friends, peers, and medical school admissions websites. What differentiates individual applicants is the way you involve yourself, the passion with which you develop your projects and the ways in which you can "sell" your experiences and skills as crucial components to becoming the "ideal" doctor.

No Cookie Cutters

Yes, all doctors will need content expertise, but each patient will have different needs that must be met by different people, each with their own approach and values. Let's say you are an oncologist. Are you going to be the type that scares the cancer away with aggression and a pushy attitude, or are you going to be the one that calmly guides a patient through? You definitely don't know the answer to that question yet, but the point is that both approaches are valid, and both will be needed by patients at different times. Though you don't know your "doctor style" yet, the more specific you can be about *how* you plan to help your patients and how your approach will allow you to address a particular need within medicine, the more convincing you will be to a committee.

Think Like an Applicant

The "checklist" of items that make a good application, such as volunteering, research, clinical experience, and teaching experience, are based on the notion that the application is somehow numerically ranked (like volunteer work will get you three points, shadowing will get you four, and the top 100 scores will get an interview). While individual schools might end up doing this to some extent in the final stages of their assessment process, there is by no means a pattern of "grading" consistent enough across schools that it should affect how you strategically plan to spend your pre-med years. Your application will be judged as part of a complete package to help admissions committees get a sense of who you are. Address it as such.

So let's break down what this application process will look like, shall we?

The application has two sets of numbers that all admissions committees will pay close attention to: your GPA (and the individual grades in each of your classes that made up that GPA) and your MCAT score (with the associated score breakdown). While these numbers won't make you, they *can* break you. I'll explain what I mean.

There is no admissions committee that will accept you only based on your scores. If you have a 4.0 GPA and 528 MCAT, but no involvement in extracurricular activities or community work, or if you cannot otherwise *show* that you are really passionate about becoming a doctor (as opposed to just great at taking exams), you might get an interview because your numbers will have caught the attention of the committee. However, you would be hard pressed to gain an acceptance. That is to say, perfect scores are enough to get your foot in the door, but probably not enough to get you a seat at the table.

If you are on the other end of the spectrum, graduating with a 2.0 GPA and a 486 MCAT score, but have a track record of commitment to your community and meaningful engagement with the medical profession, you probably won't get in either. The difference is that this student probably won't even get a chance to interview. The numbers aren't everything, but they are necessary.

Ideally, you could be that person who manages the 4.0 GPA and 528 MCAT, volunteers, shadows physicians, saves kittens from burning buildings, and still stays sane through it all. I would totally recommend being that person if you can swing it. But in case, like most of us, you are not perfect, and your pre-med journey is shaping up to be a bit of a bumpy ride, let's talk about some more realistic scenarios.

In preparation for writing this book, I spoke to members of admissions committees from schools across the country—their collective experience included elite research universities, flagship public schools, newly founded private schools, and everything in between. The most valuable piece of information I got from them is that your MCAT scores and GPA are the most important things on your application.

In a world where the number of medical school applications increases each year and more and more people are applying for the same number of spots, the admissions process increasingly becomes an exercise in splitting hairs to distinguish between similarly excellent candidates. Adcoms (admissions committees), much like the rest of the world's industries, are shifting some tasks to technology to decrease their costs and the burden on their staff. In many cases, and for an ever-increasing number of schools, much of the initial sorting of applications is being shifted to machines. Even if that is not the case for your school of choice, adcoms are BUSY. The average committee consists of 27 people who will be responsible for screening and assessing an average of 5,000+ applications between July and January, which necessitates automation of the process.

The easiest and most objective way to do that is, perhaps unsurprisingly, by screening based on your GPA and MCAT scores. Now I know that is not what anyone wants to hear, but the grim reality is that there are simply too many excellent candidates for schools to take chances on students with low scores.

If your numbers are too far below the numbers of the people a school has historically accepted, chances are you are out of the running from the start. The numbers are critical for getting your foot in the door—if you don't meet their initial threshold, you will be left out in the cold. The numbers can *break* you.

The truth is that members of admissions committees have quite a tall order to fill in having to decide which of their fantastic applicants to accept and which to turn down. All the committee members I spoke to seemed to be acutely aware of the weight of each acceptance and rejection they sent out, and what potential impact that had on the lives of the students whose applications graced their screens.

Yes, they really do want to accept you. They are human, and they realize that other humans (especially highly qualified, highly competitive, overly stressed, and largely perfectionist medical school hopefuls) sometimes make mistakes, whether academic or otherwise. They don't want to hold any of these mistakes against you, and several admissions professionals I spoke to attested to being genuinely saddened by students who presented applications that were strong across every dimension except their scores. However, as amazing, wonderful, charismatic, and kind as you are, the painful reality is that your strengths might not (read: probably won't) be enough for the person reading your application to make a case for you at a committee meeting.

Now I know what you're thinking. What about this student? Mr. I-studied-rocket-science-at-a-university-notorious-for-grade-deflation-and-worked-really-tremendously-hard-even-if-that-isn't-totally-evident-in-my-GPA. We'll call him Joe. Well, Joe probably is incredibly intelligent, as I don't know many people who complete challenging degrees at challenging universities who aren't. But that is a complete judgment call left up to each individual admissions officer, if his GPA doesn't reflect that fact. Think about it: it's not like Joe can waltz into the boardroom of Dream Medical School and convince them of his intelligence or his worth as a student in their incoming class.

Now let's say Joe's application falls into the hands of Karen, an admissions officer at Dream Medical School. Karen has had a rough morning—she forgot her coffee at home and got stuck in traffic on the way to work. She also didn't sleep well last night and is just really tired and ready for the week to be over. Now it is going to be up to Karen (and maybe a few other Karens, depending on the school and how their internal process works) to determine if Joe's application will be discussed in committee.

Note to Joe: don't make Karen's day any harder by making her come up with excuses for your below-Dream-Medical-School's-average-GPA and explain why it should be overlooked and why you should be accepted over someone whose scores speak for themselves.

If you weren't able to follow that spectacular, made-up example, the moral is this: poor grades (below the average of students that are usually admitted to your school of choice) are hard to explain away, so *you will always be better off to prioritize your numbers.*

Let's discuss how to prioritize them, practically.

Medical school hopefuls reading this book right now will fall into one of three categories:

1. Not yet begun, or are in the first half of undergrad and have a lot of space to improve their GPA

2. In the second half of undergrad and have *some* space to improve their GPA

3. Finished with undergrad and already have a closed GPA

The way to approach this will be different depending on where you are in the pre-med timeline, but there *are* ways to appeal to your target schools—no matter where you are in the timeline or what your scores currently look like. It is never too late to make yourself a strong applicant.

Just Getting Started

If you've just begun your journey, you are already ahead of the game by having picked this book, and you have plenty of opportunities to put yourself in the best possible position for getting those numbers up as high as you can. You will be faced with many, *many* choices as you navigate your first two years of college, and what each of them will ultimately boil down to is *how you will spend your time.*

Selecting Your Major

Every choice, from the major you will pursue, to the clubs you will join, to the social network you will build, will exert different demands on your time and energy. Making the right selections for yourself early on will set you up for success, whether you end up applying to medical school or not. In this section, since we are discussing keeping those scores up to maximize your chances of receiving an invitation to interview, we will chat about the process of selecting your major.

When selecting your major, the most important thing to remember is to choose something that really interests you and that you can be successful in. After all, this is probably the single subject to which you will dedicate the most time. If you have decided that medicine is the plan for you, then the ultimate goal of your undergraduate degree is to propel you into the medical school of your dreams. The good news? You can get into medical school having studied ANY major!

So now that you have virtually unlimited options, there are two things to think about when making your choice:

1. Without wanting to sound too cynical, I will say that you should pick a major that is manageable to fit into a busy schedule that won't require more than 50% of your credit hours dedicated solely to its completion. Now, this is not to say that the content will be easy. You are in a four-year college—that means that you will be asked to step outside your comfort zone to be successful. However, in terms of scheduling, the less demanding it is (i.e., a major that requires only three classes per semester to complete instead of five), the easier it will be for you to be successful and dedicate time to other pursuits.

2. Pick something that lends itself well to completing the pre-med requirements, or ensure that you have enough time to space out pre-med classes so that you can be successful in them.

Let's look at how this advice panned out for a few students that were kind enough to share their experiences.

Natalie is a med-school hopeful who wants to attend a flagship, public research university in her home state. She declared her major of neuroscience immediately, as one of the lucky people confident in and accurate about their interests from the second they set foot on a college campus. Her neuroscience degree also required her to complete all of the pre-med classes, both for credit and as qualifying prerequisites for all the upper-level courses in her major. This was a convenient arrangement for her because it allowed her to check items off of her two academic checklists (major and graduating from college/pre-med) with each course.

By the time Natalie reached her junior year, she was on track to finish her degree on time and only had to take two major-specific upper-level classes per semester. To reach full-time student status, she also added French and Spanish classes each semester, allowing her the flexibility to pursue her passion for foreign languages and relieve the stress of switching gears to her upper-level science courses. As languages come naturally to her, she found success in those courses with relative ease and was left ample time to study for her neuroscience exams when needed. With this schedule, she was able to be successful throughout her last two years of school without stretching herself too thin. By not attempting to major or minor in either language, she allowed herself the flexibility to drop those classes in when she needed to and didn't compromise the 4.0 GPA that would ultimately get her into medical school.

Now allow me now to introduce Anthony, a biochemistry and political science double major with a minor in medical Spanish. Unlike Natalie, Anthony's schedule was jam-packed with six classes and 18 credits for every semester he spent at his elite, liberal arts university. Managing his schedule and planning how to complete all of his coursework and still graduate on time required the strategic thinking of a game of Tetris. He was likely aiming for "impressively busy," but failed to realize the magnitude of the risk he was taking. He spent his semesters stressed, constantly struggling to balance the essays of his poli-sci courses with the grammar sets of his Spanish courses, along with the need for an in-depth understanding of his biochemistry courses. If that all sounds hard, it's because it was! Anthony graduated with a 3.42 GPA, leaving him below the averages of his goal schools.

Anthony tried to impress schools with his varied interests and show his ability to balance a heavy course load. He thought it would help set him apart from his peers.

Had Anthony managed to keep his GPA in line with the averages, then *maybe* (and it's a big maybe, which we will talk about in a minute) his multiple majors would have been impressive. However, a high GPA will *always* be impressive and cannot be argued. Because he couldn't actually know how he would perform in all of his classes and under all of the stress ahead of time, just aiming for more was not a wise move on Anthony's part. Instead, he could have taken some pressure off by picking which subject he enjoyed the most and just filling in the rest of his time with classes that interested him. The truth is, adcoms don't actually care what your undergrad major was!

Myth: More is better.

Moral: Better is better.

Natalie demonstrated that she can be academically successful in a rigorous environment—far better than Anthony, at least.

4.0 versus 3.42, it's that simple.

Sure, in Anthony's defense, he put in more *hours* at school and potentially can discuss a wider range of topics than Natalie, based on academics alone. You could also argue that he was more curious and more willing to be challenged, and that if he also only completed a single major, he too could have had a perfect, or near perfect, GPA. The problem with that logic is that if a computer is comparing them, it does not have the capacity to come to this conclusion. Even if a person is looking at the scores, you have to hope that human—who might be hungry, tired, anxious, stressed, or thinking about how he has to duck out early to go to his kid's play or to walk or his dog or literally a myriad other things—will go through the time and effort to make that argument. What's more? Anthony is betting that admissions officer will actually *want* to make that effort! I mean, after all, adcoms want to admit the strongest applicants, right? While you could try to talk yourself into thinking that Anthony maybe has what it takes, the admitting adcom is looking for people who can handle the rigor of their curriculum, and will definitely put their money on Natalie.

Now, in addition to the risk that Anthony took with his GPA, he also made a large, if less obvious, sacrifice. Remember how we said Natalie only took four classes per semester? That means she was only in class about 2–3 hours per day, leaving her about eight hours of productive time to fill in however she wanted: studying when necessary, paid work, extracurricular activities, lab work, volunteering, or taking a mental health day.

Conversely, a typical week had Anthony booked for 100 pages of reading for poli-sci, a problem set for biochem, and learning 250 vocab words for his weekly Spanish quiz on top of 5-6 hours of class daily. Trying to keep up with all of this academic work week-in and week-out left Anthony little time to commit to meaningful involvement in his extracurricular activities, especially because he knew how important it was to keep his GPA as high as possible. Now, even if the admissions officer reading Anthony's application had come to his defense and had been impressed by his breadth of studies, his curiosity, and his ability to be at least relatively successful across a range of academic course and styles of teaching, he would have moved on to the Activities portion of his application and compared it against Natalie's. Anthony did not carve out enough time in his schedule to commit to his nonacademic passions, and I guarantee it showed, starting on page three of his application. How committed was he able to be to a project, club, shadowing experience, or *whatever* while juggling all of that schoolwork? Chances are, Natalie also "beat" him on time committed alone.

Myth: Making yourself work hard throughout college will be impressive to committees and show them that you are prepared for medical school.

Moral: Work *hard* and work *smart*.

A final tidbit about working smart: You are in college! You get to arrange your schedule. You know at the beginning of the semester what your finals and midterm schedules will look like, what day of the week you will have homework due, and when you will have to write all of your 30-page term papers. Spend a few minutes at the beginning of each semester to make sure you are setting yourself up for success, and change some things around if you feel like you aren't. The same thing goes for classes in general. If you are planning to complete your pre-med requirements while you are in college, there is absolutely no reason for you to cram physics, organic chemistry, and biochemistry lab into a single semester. Doing well in pre-med classes is already hard enough. Don't make it harder on yourself than it has to be!

A Bit Further Along

For all of you Anthony types out there who read that section on GPAs and though "Alright Elisabeth, I hear you, but what if it's too late for me to get my GPA up to a competitive level for my schools?" Let's talk about your next steps.

The numbers given in the examples above are real scores, reported to me by real students for the purposes of this book. For that reason, the conclusions are also relative, meaning that a "good" or "competitive" GPA will vary depending on your goal schools. As long as your GPA falls within the range of GPAs reported by accepted students in the previous year (you can find that from the MSAR [Medical School Admissions Requirements], which I recommend buying), then chances are you will be considered for acceptance alongside your peers. Just remember the following points.

YOUR GPA MIGHT BE DIFFERENT THAN YOU THINK

As soon as you submit your application through the AMCAS portal, it takes about a month for them to verify your GPA and coursework. It is possible that your AMCAS GPA and your university-reported GPA will be different. When your GPA finally gets to the schools to which you have applied, there is a chance they will recompute your

GPA. Schools will receive academic records from thousands of schools throughout the country, and all of those schools have their own ways of reporting and computing grades—AMCAS helps them out by recomputing based on a set of published guidelines (you could even figure out yourself what your AMCAS GPA will be) to standardize some of those discrepancies. However, individual schools might have different priorities or standards for their admitted students that can be reflected in any recalculating they might do. This is especially relevant for something like grade forgiveness. For example, if you retake a class because of poor performance and the first attempt was removed from your transcript, the original grade will be included in your AMCAS GPA, even if it is not included in the GPA reported by your college. What your school will do with that attempt is, as usual, up to the individual school.

DIFFERENT SCHOOLS WEIGH SCORES DIFFERENTLY

There is incredible variation among how U.S. medical schools design their admissions process. How medical schools will look at your grades from different subjects, your overall versus your biology/chemistry/physics/math (BCPM) GPAs, and your performance across different years in college will vary tremendously from school to school *and* from year to year! So don't count yourself out just yet.

IMPROVEMENT IS ALWAYS IMPRESSIVE

If you are someone who did particularly poorly throughout your first few years in college, there is one piece of very good news: you have loads of room for improvement! If you continue to do well academically as you progress through your college years, adcoms will be confident that even if you had a tough time adjusting to college, they will meet you at the end of an upward trajectory.

Myth: Having one bad grade in a pre-med class will disqualify you from attending your goal schools.

Moral: Medical schools are looking at trends in academic performance as much as they are individual grades.

Degree Already Completed

If you are already out of undergrad and cannot improve your GPA, there are a few key things to think about. First, the gap year(s) you are currently in give you an opportunity to amass experiences that will make you stand out on things apart from your GPA. The remaining portions of your application are likely stronger than those of your competitors, which is fantastic news! As for your GPA, think carefully about what kinds of schools you are interested in applying to, keeping in mind the following:

1. If your GPA is still significantly below your goals, it might be time to think about a Post-Bac or Master's program. This is a great (albeit expensive) opportunity for you to show schools that you are on an upward trajectory and can handle rigorous graduate coursework. Again, the goal is to indicate that you

can handle the academic challenges you will face in medical school.

2. If your GPA is slightly below the range of accepted applicants for that school, assess your MCAT scores. Are they above the average enough to "cancel out" lower scores? Don't try to answer this yourself! Contact the schools you are interested in by phone and ask about how they will specifically be assessing your GPA and MCAT scores. If you have not yet taken your MCAT, use your GPA as a benchmark to help you determine what a goal score is for you.

Myth: Graduating with a low GPA disqualifies you from becoming a doctor.

Moral: It is never too late to show medical schools that you can handle their curriculum, and there are many academic opportunities you can pursue post-graduation to do so!

What Med School Wants You to Consider

Like I said, however, the numbers are only enough to get your foot in the door. Stellar grades alone will not lead directly to your acceptance on their own.

As we have mentioned multiple times before, the intent of the application to medical school is to prove to an admissions committee, based on your passion projects and extracurricular involvement, that you are:

1. Mature

2. Committed

3. Knowledgeable enough about the field

They want to believe when you say that you want to be a doctor. The responsibility admissions committees have to ensure you know what you are getting yourself into makes a lot of sense when you consider the following.

Expense

Medical school is an arduous and expensive commitment, followed by even more arduous years of residency and fellowship programs. You could fill out the application when you are 22 years old, but what you are really committing to is a process of learning (and paying for a lot of that learning) until you are 32 years old!

Investment

Schools invest a lot of money in training and educating you while you are in their care. As unbelievable as this will sound given the exorbitant costs of tuition, medical schools are subsidizing the cost of your education through federal grants and endowments. They want to make sure that they are getting their money's worth when they accept you, and that you won't decide to flake out halfway through the program. This is also why they weigh MCAT scores so heavily. In order to become a practicing physician and for them to legally graduate you, you must pass the United States Medical Licensing Examination (USMLE), known colloquially as Step 1. Your ability to succeed on the exam is highly correlated with your performance on the MCAT, so they really look to your score as a sign of your ability to succeed in the future.

Commitment

In-state institutions are especially subsidized by state governments because individuals are more likely to work in areas where they were educated. States are quite literally paying for their future local doctors to get an education. That means they can't afford to have you get your degree and skip off to run a private hospital or become a med tech consultant. They have to be sure that you are actually committed to the practice of medicine down the line.

Now, of course, adcoms can be wrong when they make judgments about applicants. Plenty of people go off into other careers, using the legitimacy of their newly minted degrees to gain traction in the workforce. But the point of the application is to convince them that you are at least no more likely to do that than the Average Joe.

Orient your time around highlighting to the adcoms that you are mature, committed, and knowledgeable about the field of medicine, all the while prioritizing your academic performance, and you will be a strong candidate by the time you are ready to apply.

THE PRIMARY APPLICATION | 3

The primary application is the first official communication you will have with the medical schools to which you will apply. The pieces that make up the primary will be sent centrally to one of three databases: AACOMAS (American Association of Colleges of Osteopathic Medicine) if you are applying to osteopathic medical schools, TMDSAS (Texas Medical & Dental Schools Application Service) if you are applying to public medical schools in the Texas system, and AMCAS (American Medical College Application Service) for all other U.S. medical schools. These centralized systems will then forward the pieces of your application to the individual medical schools that you specify. You won't begin to have direct contact with individual medical schools until after they have received a completed, processed, and verified primary application for you from one of these central databases.

While the applications are similar in that they will request *essentially* the same information, they are (surprise, surprise) just different enough that you can't copy and paste between them if you are applying to schools that require different applications.

The main differences are:

1. The TMDSAS application requires three essays, while the AMCAS and the AACOMAS require one each (everything is bigger in Texas).

2. Through the AMCAS system, you can decide which recommendation letters get sent to which schools, while for the other two systems, all letters collected will be sent to all schools.

3. The main application questions for each database, which we will refer to throughout this book as "the personal statement," are just different enough in length and prompt that you cannot copy and paste between them.

Be aware of these differences and the additional finessing your application will need if you plan to apply to schools that are served by more than one central system. As AMCAS is by far the most commonly used of the three databases, details discussed here will be specific to the AMCAS application. However, the key themes discussed will be pertinent to applications flowing through any of the systems.

ACTION ITEMS: SUBMIT DAY 1

While you will have the option to add information to your primary application for the entire length of the application season, the best and easiest thing you can do to improve your chances of turning the application into an interview is to *submit your primary application as early as possible* (when the system opens, if you can).

The application will accept submissions on June 1 for applicants intending to matriculate to medical school in August of the following year. However, the system itself opens one month earlier, on May 1, allowing you to start inputting information so that you are actually able to click the submit button on Day 1.

If you have a pre-med advisor worth their salt, they will have told you to aim for submission on June 1. If not, let me say it again: Submit. Your. Application. On. June. 1. This recommendation is in place because the timing of your submission will be instrumental for the remainder of your application process, and may mean the difference between an acceptance and a rejection. Most schools operate rolling admissions, which means that they read applications, invite interviewees, and extend admissions offers *as they come in!* That means that if a school has planned, for example, 100 interview slots to fill between August and December, an applicant who submitted his application in June will be considered for all 100 of those slots.

By contrast, an applicant who has submitted in October, around the last date for submitting the primary application, may only be considered for 25 of those spots. This isn't because the late applicant is any less qualified than the early one. It just means, quite simply, that those 75 spots no longer exist. The interview dates have come and gone, and other people who were organized enough to get their applications in before you were invited to go on them.

You are now in a pool of applicants competing for 75% fewer spots because you delayed your submission. You basically just made the process *more* competitive for yourself. Not your best move. That is not to say, of course, that you are destined to fail if you do delay the submission of your primary application. Those remaining seats will still get filled by someone. However, in this application game, there are too many qualified applicants to begin with. You are better off improving your chances as much as you can, especially with something as simple as submitting on time.

Chris from Colorado says, "I had this notion that neuroticism over a week or two delay wouldn't make or break my application, but having seen how long the committee reviews every application on the other side of the submit button and the sometimes arbitrary nature of how qualified applications are distinguished from the pile, I now believe that *when* you send in a completed application is one of the few factors that applicants have actual control over at the application stage."

Additionally, if you are planning on submitting to a school through an Early Decision Program, make sure you are keeping track of those deadlines and similarly taking advantage of the opportunity to submit as early as possible.

THE PRIMARY APPLICATION

The primary application consists of eight parts. They are briefly described here, but we will go into more detail about the MCAT, Activities List, Personal Statement, Letters of

Recommendation, and School List in greater detail in later chapters.

Demographics

You will be asked to answer questions about identifying and contact information, biographical and parental information, and details about your childhood. You will also be asked if you come from a disadvantaged socioeconomic background, if you grew up in a medically underserved area, or if you felt you had other demographic or socioeconomic challenges that impacted your journey to medical school. Now I know what you're thinking: *Why are medical schools so nosy? Having to provide so much information and so many details about my life seems pretty intrusive.* I have to say, I totally agree. However, it is the only way for medical school admissions committees to get a sense of who you are as a whole, including your childhood, parental, socioeconomic, and demographic details. This information will give them a sense of what environment you are from, what challenges you faced, and what unique perspectives you will bring to the practice of medicine. Medical school admissions committees are charged not only with selecting which college graduates will be turned into stellar physicians, but also with the more practical, short-term goal of building a matriculating class of students that can help one another grow, develop, and greatly benefit a national patient population that is constantly becoming more diverse. These questions may seem intrusive, but they are intended to help adcoms determine which students will be able to offer diverse perspectives across multiple dimensions, and thus help schools to graduate better, more informed doctors.

Then the obvious next question is, is *not* being disadvantaged a disadvantage? Fortunately, the answer is no. Having come from a more comfortable or affluent financial background comes with its own unique perspectives, including perhaps the opportunity to have travelled, done volunteer work abroad, or engaged in other activities not available to someone who spent her undergraduate years working to pay tuition. Again, the intent of adcoms here is to create a class full of diverse perspectives on the complicated topics their students will face. As long as you answer these questions in an honest and compelling way, you will be just fine.

Disciplinary action

There will also be space on the primary application for you to specify whether you have ever had disciplinary action taken against you, whether you have ever committed a felony or misdemeanor, or whether you have been given something other than an honorable discharge as a military veteran. On the AMCAS, you will be given 1,300 characters to address the situation if your answer to any of these questions is "yes." While having to write anything in this section of the application is less than ideal, it will not keep you from getting into medical school. Make sure to use the available space to explain what happened, what you learned from the situation, how you grew, and what you would do differently if given the opportunity or if you were to face a similar set of circumstances in the future. The goal of your entire application to medical school is to show that you are mature enough to handle the responsibility of a medical school education, and this section is no different. Should you need to address this part of the application, be completely honest with your schools and indicate that you take responsibility for the mistakes you have made.

I'm going to say this again, in case you skimmed over it before: DO NOT LIE about disciplinary action! That includes failing to disclose any relevant information. You never know what information might cross the paths of the people of your committee—not to mention what they could find on their own by quickly searching the Internet for your name. While having disciplinary action against you will not cost you your admission, lying about it most definitely will.

ACADEMIC RECORD

Your academic record will contain the courses you took, the dates you took them, and the grades you received. If your school allows you to access this online, then the information is really simple to just download and use as needed. If not, make sure you give yourself and your school plenty of time to get a copy so that you can forward it along to AMCAS and ultimately your medical schools of choice.

But it doesn't end there.

In addition to forwarding your transcripts directly from all of the academic institutions you have attended, you will also be required to manually input all of the information from your transcript into the application itself. AMCAS will ask you to copy over the number of credits, date of completion, and final grade of every course you ever took in an undergraduate, post-bac, or post-grad program. Now, if you are crazy like me you may be able to do this from memory without a transcript, and I offer you my deepest sympathies. If not, make sure you prepare for needing this.

An important note about this part of the application is that just the process of inputting the information itself is incredibly time consuming. Don't scoff at this. It is one of the reasons the application system opens for edits an entire month before it opens for submissions. Completing the entire primary in one sitting is simply not going to be an option, due in no small part to the manual labor associated with inputting this information.

It is also important to note that your medical schools will not see the same information about yourself that you do. When you send your transcripts to any of these three central databases, they will recompute your grades according to a standardized set of regulations. For example, if your undergraduate institution didn't have – or + grades, AMCAS will recompute the GPA you will see to distinguish between, let's say, a B and a B+. Similarly, if your college or university had policies that allowed you to "cover" a poor grade in the event you retook the class and scored better, that grade *will* show up in your AMCAS-calculated GPA, even if it didn't show up on your undergraduate transcript. This recalculation process is intended to standardize the information that medical schools receive, so they can more easily compare applicants who completed different programs.

But that is not all. Your GPA might be calculated *again* by each of your medical schools, in accordance with their guidelines. For example, some schools may discount your freshman and sophomore grades if they believe that everyone deserves some time to adjust to college. Others may weigh your BCPM GPA more heavily than your overall GPA, if they feel that performance in those courses is more indicative of students' success in their curriculum than overall academic performance.

The bottom line is that you probably don't know what your GPA is for the purposes of the medical school application, so all you can do is perform as well as you can in your circumstances (and there isn't much value to obsessively calculating it, either).

MCAT

The scores from all the times you have taken the MCAT will show up in your primary application and be made visible for the schools to which you are applying. Again, how each school will assess these scores will depend on the policies of each individual institution. For example, if you have taken the test more than once, schools will make their own decisions about whether they will take the highest score, lowest score, most recent score, first score, or an average of the available results. Schools may also give differential weight to individual sections, likely informed by how they feel scores on individual sections are indicative of students' performance in that specific academic environment. Ultimately, schools will use this section of the application to determine whether or not you can take standardized tests. After all, a medical student who can't pass the USMLE won't become a doctor.

An important thing to note about the MCAT section of the application is that, along with the letters of recommendation, it does not have to be complete for you to submit your primary on time. However, you will need to have a set of MCAT scores for your whole application to be considered "complete" by the schools that will be looking at it, so if you submit without a score, you better be sure you are planning to get that hole filled as soon as possible.

Activities List

This is the portion of the application where you will get to highlight your soft skills as demonstrated by the way you have spent your time leading up to the application. These soft skills include all the things that we talked about adcoms looking for in future doctors, like maturity, empathy, grit, compassion, patience, the ability and willingness to serve patients, and many more. You may list up to 15 activities in a variety of categories. You will then designate three of these as your "most valuable experiences" and get more space to write about them and explain what you did, what you learned, and how they impacted you. When selecting your "most valuable experiences," you will want to select at least one clinical experience to highlight your interest in medical school and the opportunities it will afford you. Other than that quick rule of thumb, you have plenty of latitude in how to lay this section out.

Personal Statement

The personal statement is the largest piece of writing in the primary application. In the personal statement, you will explain why you want to be a doctor and convince adcoms that you have what it takes to make it through the program. This is also an opportunity for you to add a third dimension to the otherwise flat representation of you as a set of numbers and accomplishments.

Letters of Recommendation

AMCAS will allow you to submit up to 10 letters of recommendation and to determine which letters you will send to which schools. You will have to look at the requirements of each of the schools you intend to apply to in order to determine what types of recommendations they want to see in support of your application. For example, some schools may require letters of support from science professors, research advisors, or volunteer supervisors. It will be your responsibility to ensure that your application meets the admissions criteria for each of the schools you are interested in. Failing to send schools the right number or type of recommendation letter is a sure way to shoot yourself in the foot while racing to the finish line.

Again, the letters of recommendation do not have to be submitted for you to submit your portion of the application for verification. However, you will have to list the names and contact information of your recommenders. Schools won't look at your application until all of those pieces of information have been submitted, so it will be to your benefit to ensure that those are submitted sooner rather than later.

School List

The final pages of your application will include a list of all the schools to which you have applied. The creation of the list will be one of the most time-consuming pieces of your application process, and is likely to be one of the most impactful for the state of your candidacy. The fact that this list of schools will be available for all adcoms to see can also be an important wrench in this process. For example, if you write your personal statement about your passion for primary care but apply only to major research institutions, it might call your credibility into question. Of course, adcoms are not necessarily interested in scrutinizing your application in that level of depth, but trying to avoid inconsistencies like that can only help you throughout this process.

As soon as you have all these parts of the application ready to go, you will submit your application to one (or more than one, depending on what your school list looks like) centralized database for processing and verification. Be aware that you will also need to have the fees at this time. It will then take about a month for your application to be processed, verified, and distributed to the schools you have specified. As soon as that happens, you will be done with the primary application to medical school and will be waiting for requests to submit your secondary applications from each individual school.

Here it is. The chapter you've all been dreading…or the chapter on the thing you will eventually be dreading if you haven't completed it already: the Medical College Admissions Test (MCAT)…dun dun dun. So let's get some facts about this thing out in the open.

The MCAT is a seven-hour-and-thirty-minute long, standardized, multiple-choice examination that is developed and administered by the AAMC (Association of American Medical Colleges).

It is made up of four sections: Chemical and Physical Foundations of Biological Systems; Critical Analysis and Reasoning Skills; Biological and Biochemical Foundations of Living Systems; and Psychological, Social, and Biological Foundations of Behavior. I will refer to them colloquially for the rest of this book because, let's face it, those names are a mouthful. Chemical and Physical Foundations of Biological Systems becomes Chem/Phys; Critical Analysis and Reasoning Skills becomes CARS, which is essentially reading comprehension; Biological and Biochemical Foundations of Living Systems becomes Bio/Biochem; and Psychological, Social, and Biological Foundations of Behavior becomes Psych/Soc.

Here is the order of events for your Test Day:

Section	Time
Examinee agreement	8 minutes
Tutorial (optional)	10 minutes
Chem/Phys • 44 passage-based questions, 15 standalone, non-passage-related questions for a total of 59	95 minutes
Break (optional)	10 minutes
CARS • 53 passage-based questions	90 minutes
Mid-exam (lunch) break (optional)	30 minutes
Bio/Biochem • 44 passage-based questions, 15 standalone, non-passage-related questions for a total of 59	95 minutes
Break (optional)	10 minutes
Psych/Soc • 44 passage-based questions, 15 standalone, non-passage-related questions for a total of 59	95 minutes
Void question (where you get asked if you want to pretend like you didn't just spend the last 7 hours of your life in a room full of stressed-out people testing)	5 minutes
Satisfaction Survey (optional)	5 minutes
Total content time	6 hours, 15 minutes
Total seated time	7 hours, 30 minutes

- Scores for each section range from 118 to 132, putting the maximum score at 528 and the scaled median at 500, or 125 per section.

- The basic registration fee for the MCAT is $315, which covers the cost of you sitting for the exam and for the AAMC to distribute your scores to all of the schools to which you will apply. Late registration or rescheduling your test will lead to additional fees.

- The AAMC will only allow you to take the MCAT up to three times per testing year, four times during a consecutive two-year period, and only seven times in your life. Hopefully you won't be looking at numbers that high, but it is available as an option if necessary.

- Yes, schools will see the scores from *every one* of your attempts, unless you cancel the scores within the five-minute void window you are given post-exam to cancel the scores.

- If you cancel your score, the schools you apply to won't even know you went to test that day—it will be like it never happened. Well, almost…you won't get a refund of your money if you cancel the test.

- If you are scheduled for a test and don't show up to take it, there will obviously be no score to report, but it will count toward your lifetime limit.

- The breaks given between subjects are *technically* optional. But let me say again, in case you missed it in my earlier iterations, that this test is SEVEN hours long. Don't be a hero. Take the damn breaks.

- Scores break down as follows:
  - ° Top 10% of testers have a scaled total score between 514 and 528
  - ° Top 25% of testers have a scaled total score between 508 and 513
  - ° Top 50% of testers have a scaled total score between 500 and 507
  - ° Bottom 50% of testers score a 499 or below

The MCAT requires you to have a breadth of fundamental knowledge and the skills to apply that knowledge to the novel information introduced to you in the question stems—that is, stuff that you didn't have to study for the test, but that you will be expected to be able to reason through based on stuff you *did* have to study for the test. The relevant subjects are two semesters each of Biology, General Chemistry, Physics, and Organic Chemistry, and one semester each of Biochemistry, Psychology, and Sociology.

Let that sink in for just a second.

That is 11 classes worth of material!

The MCAT requires more content knowledge than any other test that you have taken in your life (before you actually get to medical school, of course), and will be more impactful than any other test you have taken as well. (Really puts all those midterms and finals you've been stressing about into perspective huh?)

Now I consider myself a bit of an MCAT expert, having worked as a Kaplan MCAT tutor for over three years and having helped hundreds of students over that time navigate the stressful and overwhelming process of studying for this monster of an exam. Adding that to the fact that I took the test twice myself (the second attempt taught me that I am apparently masochistic and enjoy putting immense stress on myself for little potential gain, but more on his later), I have spent probably thousands of hours of my short life thinking and stressing and studying and trying to talk myself out of medical school over this exam! Like I said, expert.

In all of my wisdom on this thrilling topic, I am going to walk you through some frequently asked questions that will affect when, how, and with what goal you should embark on your personal MCAT journey.

When to Take the Test

You will see that as you go through the application process, you will begin thinking about time in three-month chunks, during which you will have to complete hefty tasks like prepping for and taking the MCAT. So while in the process of deciding when to take this test, you not only have to think about whether you are actually available on the day of the test itself, but also about how much time you can afford to clear (from school, work, other obligations) in the months leading up to doomsday to prepare for it.

The date you intend to test has the potential to affect everything from your academic schedule to the cycle in which you will matriculate. In the following section, I will present all the potential test dates to help you work through which is best for you.

Your timing for taking the MCAT will depend on when you want to apply to medical school and how much flexibility you have in your schedule for studying. As we have mentioned before, you should aim to submit your application in June the year before you are planning to begin medical school, so all of these potential test dates will be discussed assuming this as your plan.

MAY / BEGINNING OF JUNE

If you intend to submit your application with the first batch of applicants, which I *absolutely* recommend, then the *latest date you can test and not have it delay your application is May 31* of that same year. This is because you upload your primary application to AMCAS, the central database that will verify your transcripts and then send the application out to the list of schools you have specified. That month-long verification process can act as a buffer for MCAT preparation—because schools won't get your application until July 1 anyway, you can delay your MCAT so that the scores are also ready on that date. The farther into June you push the test date, the more your application will be delayed. If you are able to get it done by the middle of the month, that slight delay in the application will not be the end of the world. However, the goal is to apply as early as possible, so you definitely won't have a lot of cushion here.

THE GOOD

- No delay to your application (assuming you get the remainder of your application submitted on time)

- Maximum amount of time available to study

- If you are in school when you take the MCAT, this will give you a few weeks after the end of your finals to dedicate solely to MCAT prep

THE BAD

Because avoiding a delay to your application depends upon you being ready to submit the rest of your application on that June 1 date, preparing to take the MCAT while also preparing your primary will require a bit of a balancing act on your end.

"MacGyvering" this last-minute test date into a successful strategy will require you to take a big risk: applying without knowing your MCAT score. How important the score will be in determining your list of schools will depend in part on your temperament and on the strength of the rest of your application, but chances are it will have at least a bit of an impact.

THE WORKAROUND

To help you balance the completion of the primary application (read: personal statement and activities list) with the completion of the MCAT portion of your application you want to stretch both of these out as much as possible. Do *not* plan to "cram" for the MCAT or to crank out your primary in a few days. Chances are you will end up with a subpar product and present a less-than-ideal version of yourself to adcoms. This is absolutely not the time to drop the ball. So then what *should* you do? If you are planning to test at the end of May or beginning of June, you want to plan to at least have the bulk of the primary application out of the way before you start studying. Speaking from personal experience, both studying for the MCAT and preparing your primary statement are time- and mind-consuming processes, and you will be much better off if you manage to separate them.

To avoid the stress that comes with applying without knowing your score, there is a slight life hack you can take advantage of to get the best of both worlds: maximum time to study for the MCAT and the flexibility to design your school list after receiving your score (although it does still require you to have your primary application ready on time). On June 1, submit the primary application through AMCAS, but list only one school. This school should be one that you are reasonably going to apply to no matter what—Harvard Medical School for the optimist, your state or linkage school for the realist. When you do this, you will have applied to medical school and paid your application fee ($170 for the first school for 2019), and AMCAS will begin the month-long process of verifying your application. While AMCAS is processing, you will get your score back and can refine your goal school list and add to the system. *The process of adding schools is then practically automatic and will not delay your application in any way.* Effectively, this workaround allows you to see your score before applying, without delaying the time at which your schools will receive and begin assessing your application.

Now of course, there is a risk associated with this "hack," which is that your score is not competitive enough to apply to schools you would be happy attending—or to medical school at all. *That means that you have to be prepared to withdraw your application at this point and to forfeit the time and money you spent submitting the primary.*

ADDED BONUS

Apart from giving you extra time to prepare for the MCAT, this apply-to-one-school-first method can act as a financial buffer as well, giving you up to four or five extra weeks to save some additional money for the (admittedly quite expensive) application process.

March and April

If all of that last-minute decision making I described in the last section sounds overwhelming to you, or if you already know that you will start studying early and would like this test out of your life as soon as possible, then the March and April test dates might be ideal for you.

THE GOOD

You will have plenty of time to get your scores back before either making a list of schools to apply to or deciding whether or not you intend to apply this cycle.

These dates give you the flexibility to either delay your test until May if you're not prepared by the time your test date rolls around, or to retake the test in May if you are unhappy with your score (assuming you keep studying even after you have taken the test, in anticipation of this possibility).

THE BAD

If you are in school (i.e., you are planning on taking this test in the spring of either your sophomore, junior, or senior year), you will have to balance your classwork and extracurricular schedule with the studying for the MCAT.

JANUARY / FEBRUARY

January is a month when most people, whether they are in school or post-grad, will have had the most time to dedicate to studying and preparing for this exam.

THE GOOD

Most colleges and universities give the entire month off to their students, and almost everyone has at least a few days off in December in light of the holiday season. You can take advantage of this time as dedicated study days in anticipation of your test date.

THE BAD

Right before January comes December—a month often filled with finals for those of you that are still in school. For those who have already graduated, it's a time often full of work deadlines, family time, holiday parties, tinsel-decorated trees, and flavored hot chocolates that will call to you in those weeks when it feels like midnight at 4 PM. I have seen *so* many people (myself included) plan to be productive during the off days in December, only to watch the clock strike midnight on January 1 and realize they don't know the first thing about stoichiometric equations.

THE WORKAROUND

If you know that testing during these months will work for you, start preparing early (I'm talking the summer before) *especially if you are in school!* It is incredibly challenging to balance academics and MCAT prep when both are vying for the same hours, attention, and brain space. What's more? You can't sacrifice one for the other. Both are incredibly important, and I can guarantee that in October, the biochemistry midterm you have next week will always take precedence over the MCAT you registered for three months from now. The earlier you start, the more feasible it will be for you to pull this off.

June, July, August, and September

When I say test in June, I am talking about June the year **before** you will apply to medical school. If you aren't planning on testing until July (much less August or September) of your application year, you are already behind the curve.

THE GOOD

If you intend to test the summer before the summer you apply to medical school, then congratulations! You are ahead of the curve! August dates are by far the most popular because students tend to use the entire preceding summer for studying, prep courses, and practice tests.

THE BAD

Planning to spend an entire summer studying for the MCAT sounds like a fabulous idea until it's the middle of July and you're still doing it. Keep in mind that the process of studying for a test like this is a marathon, and a lonely one at that. Plus, if you are still in school, your MCAT-filled summer will be followed by an academic-filled semester.

THE WORKAROUND

The earlier in the summer you test, the less time you will have to study, but the more time you will have on the back end to recharge. Consider what combination of study-vs.-rest time is most feasible for you to pull off (and before you even think it, I can guarantee that all-study and no-rest time is probably *not* the best answer).

Know Yourself

So I've gone through some pros and cons for testing on various dates throughout the year. However, the benefit of these considerations comes only from you knowing *yourself* well enough to pick out which scenario pertains to you and therefore might impact your decision in the best way. For example, before I set the date for my MCAT, I also had to think about what the preceding weeks and months were going to look like and whether my date was feasible for the score I was aiming for. Here is what I knew about myself before embarking on the "logistics" portion of the planning process:

- It takes me a few days to get myself into the swing of a new routine, but when I do, I am a marathon studier…

- …who also gets distracted pretty easily.

That information, along with a finals schedule that ended at the beginning of May and the knowledge that I would need a substantial mental break between the MCAT and my first semester of senior year, put me at a July 8 date. Going in, I also allowed myself some flexibility, knowing that if the beginning of July rolled around and I needed a few extra weeks to study it wouldn't be the end of the world. The good news is that you can take the MCAT whenever you want to. You get to arrange everything about this schedule, including for which application cycle you are testing. To plot your test schedule to your advantage, you need to design a plan based on what you know about yourself. Can you study during the holidays? Are you intuitively able to be successful on standardized tests? Are you a slow reader? Is extra practice something that you need to budget time for? Do you study better in the morning or in the afternoon?

Let's use an example person here: Ankit is a college senior in Ohio who registered in November for an April test date. He began his study plan in December, and by the beginning of January, Ankit was stressed. Due to his work and school schedule, Ankit was only managing to get in about two hours of studying per day. After three weeks of studying for the MCAT, he had barely finished up a review of only his biochemistry book. As he watched the MCAT countdown on his phone decrease by the day, he felt overwhelmed. Why did it suddenly seem like he had never heard of biology before in his life? He was getting As and Bs in his science classes, so what gives? Well, something interesting happens emotionally when you are studying for an exam that you have only heard bad things about, and it is no fun: everything you have ever known about these subjects seems to fly right out of your head.

If I haven't convinced you yet that the MCAT is a pretty big deal and should be approached with a plan, here is a fun fact: when we conducted a survey of medical students across the country and asked them to give us the advice they wish they had when they were pre-meds, 86% of them gave an answer related to the MCAT.

A few answers were in the ballpark of "Take your time studying for the MCAT":

> *"Studying for the MCAT was the most stressful part of the application process, I think partly because I had other commitments in addition to studying. I think it would be preferable to extend the amount of time I was studying for the exam to reduce the stress."*

> *"It was okay to push everything back. I felt so much pressure to finish by a certain timeline and I wish I would have realized that having more time to study could have improved my MCAT by a few points, which could have made all the difference."*

A few other answers subtly suggest you prepare for the test while you are in undergrad:

> *"Take great notes in every class that will be useful for MCAT review and go in to office hours/get a tutor if feeling at all unsure of harder concepts."*

> *"Studying for the MCAT many years out of undergrad was wildly stressful. I would make sure to give myself more time to study for my exam and be more gentle with myself. It takes a long time to relearn (or learn for the first time in some cases) the material for the exam."*

And one respondent was not so subtle:

> *"Study for the MCAT in undergraduate —not after graduating."*

How to Prepare for the MCAT

Now I know you're thinking "Fine, I get it. Start studying for the MCAT early. Take it while I'm still in school. Give myself a lot of time to prepare. All of that seems easy enough, but how do I actually prepare to prepare? It all seems overwhelming and I don't know where to start."

Fabulous question!

Okay, so let's say you registered to take the test on April 13. You know what your school schedule is, and you know what your work schedule is, and you know that sometimes you're not amazing at keeping a schedule, so you will reasonably be able to commit four hours a day to studying for this test. The next step is to figure out how many weeks of studying that will amount to. The AAMC estimates that it takes the average student anywhere between 300 and 500 hours of studying to be successful on the test, but figuring out how long *you* will need to get a score that *you* are happy with will require a few steps to calculate on your part.

Be Honest

Being successful on the MCAT requires two distinct but related skill sets. The first is your understanding of the content that the exam is testing. This is that 11 classes-worth of material, and how well you understand (note this is different from how well you can *memorize*) the material taught in the introductory pre-med courses. About 30% of the questions in the Chem/Phys, Bio/Biochem, and Psych/Soc sections will be questions testing pure content knowledge. For the other 70% of the questions on the exam, you will need an additional skill, the mastery of the MCAT *process*. This entails taking the relevant content you know and the relevant details from the passage or question stem, and mixing them together to arrive at the correct answer… oh, and doing it all in about a minute and a half per question.

Now what you just read is a bit of an exercise in that "know yourself" thing I keep mentioning. If you read those last few sentences and thought "No prob," then you must be pretty solid at standardized testing. If thinking about having to do all of that analytical problem solving in a time-pressurized testing environment made you sweat, you might want to consider investing in some test prep resources to help you build the skills you will need.

Figure Out What You Know and What You Don't Know

Here's how.

TAKE A FULL-LENGTH DIAGNOSTIC EXAM

The first thing you want to do before you start your test prep, whether you do it on your own or with the help of a test prep company or tutor, is to take a full-length diagnostic exam. AAMC offers these for purchase online, or one may be given for free through your school. Regardless, you want to take a full-length test under test prep conditions. In other words, take breaks only when they are scheduled, use up all of the time, and try to work through a question even when it seems intimidating or tricky. It will be long and quite painful, but you have to power through, if for no other reason than to scare yourself into really getting serious about this studying thing.

CELEBRATE

Congrats, you just finished your first full-length test! Please celebrate with your favorite guilty pleasure—trust me, you will need mini-celebrations throughout this process if you are going to make it through unscathed. Now you want to sit down with a copy of the questions, along with a copy of the answer key and the answers you gave. You need to assess *every single question,* with particular emphasis on the ones that are incorrect. Students tend to get questions wrong because they need to shore up one of the two skills I mentioned above: either your content knowledge isn't there (totally understandable as a starting point, especially if you haven't taken a general biology class since first semester freshman year), or you misunderstood/didn't completely read/didn't get to answer the question. Take this time to figure out what you know and what you don't. Make a list here and plan to prioritize your weakest subjects first.

FIGURE OUT YOUR BEST STUDY HABITS

Think back on all the information you have amassed about yourself over the years: How do you learn best, from a video or a textbook? Do you take notes or just listen? Do you talk yourself through information, then take quizzes on the information you just learned? The MCAT study process is *not* the time to rock the boat on effective study techniques. Do whatever you have always done—it clearly worked enough to get you to this point!

Use all of the information you just spelled out for yourself to build a study plan that pinpoints your areas of weakness, exploits your strengths and skills, and prepares you to be as efficient and successful as possible.

GET INTO THE TESTMAKER'S HEAD

This test is called a "standardized" test for a reason! All of the questions and all of the passages follow a fairly similar format that can be identified and exploited. If you sign up for a prep class, the company you register with will have done the work and will be able to tell you some tips and tricks. However, if you choose not to go that route, you can always try to figure some of the info out on your own. Again, know how willing and able you will be to go at that process by yourself, and how successful you will be if you don't. Trying to get into the AAMC's head to figure out what questions will be asked is not a particularly challenging task, especially if you are naturally good at standardized tests and have a lot of time to study. However, know that most of the people you will be competing against will have committed either the time or the money to a tutor or company to gain some of these insights, and you may be behind the curve if you don't do the same.

A WORD OF ENCOURAGEMENT

If you are currently thinking about or studying for the MCAT, I know what an incredibly overwhelming process it can be. Even if your diagnostic was not where you wanted it to be, there is good news: being successful on the MCAT is a *skill*, much like running a marathon or learning how to play the piano. Fortunately, it is a skill that can usually be learned much faster and with less training than either of those. No matter where your starting point is, it is possible to be as successful as you want to be on this exam, as long as you put in the time and effort to train.

What the Scores Mean

So now when I'm testing, I know how to organize myself to start studying, and I know what skills I need to build. How do I know if I'm happy with my scores? How will schools use them to assess my candidacy?

About a month after you take your MCAT, you will get your score report back. It will include two sets of numbers—your weighted score and your percentile range—for each of the four distinct sections and for the test overall. The first will be a function of how many questions you answered correctly on a particular section and on the test overall. The second will depend on how successful everyone else taking the test was at answering those same questions on those same passages.

Your goal score, or the score to aim for as you go through this test, will depend on the schools to which you intend to apply. A good rule of thumb is a competitive applicant will have scored a 510 (81st percentile) for all medical schools, and a 517 (95th percentile) for elite medical schools.

Should You Retake the Test?

Well, lucky for all of you, I made the mistake of doing this when it wasn't necessary. I will talk about it in the following chapter so that you don't have to do the same.

TAKING THE MCAT...AGAIN | 5

When I got my MCAT scores back, I was elated. Well, to be honest, first, I was nauseous. It took me about 25 minutes to actually muster up the courage to type in my login information and click the "See my scores" button. I was on vacation with my family at the time and had returned from the beach to the hotel to check them on what seemed to be the world's slowest Wi-Fi. The sweat on my palms left prints on the laptop touchpad. Besides the fact that it was mid-August and the temperature hovered somewhere in the high 90s, I was about to check *the* score, the numbers that would, I was convinced, determine my entire professional future. But anyway, back to being elated.

My joy lasted about 15 seconds, about the time that it took for my eyes to first focus on the overall score, then shift to the left where the percentile was showing, then mentally benchmark this against my target. When all of that was over, confusion settled in. There were broad questions that no admissions or pre-professional counselor would try to answer before my scores were released: What does this mean for my list of schools? Should I alter my targets? Could my application potentially be ready for submission earlier than I thought? But then, something really interesting happened. As I sat on that hotel couch and looked more thoroughly at my score report, I noticed something a little bit odd. Despite an overall score that I was happy with, the breakdown of the individual section scores revealed a weakness in my understanding of the material that I was sure would give me a run for my money at some point down the line.

I should preface this by saying that I majored in biology in college. I had convinced myself that if so many students taking the MCAT had taken only the pre-med requirements for biology, that is, the two semesters of introductory courses, then surely my three years of advanced courses on the subject would put me ahead of the curve. (Note to self: be wary in the future of "strategic" thinking like this.) Using this knowledge, I dropped the Bio/Biochem section of the MCAT to the last priority in my study plan. I dedicated the smallest number of days to the material, completed the least number of practice tests, and generally allowed it to be my "stress free" subject. If you take one thing from this book, let it be that my strategy was definitely not the way to go. It's the MCAT, and you don't get to have a stress-free subject.

As you may have guessed already, my score in this section was low enough that it had the potential to, in the words of my pre-professional advisor "…call into question my ability to keep up with the rigor of science-based material that I would be called upon to learn in medical school, and statistically, significantly diminish the chances that my Step 1 score will be competitive enough to place into a residency." I was floored, but put on my bravest face. "Okay, so I take it again," I remember saying matter-of-factly. "Well," she replied, "I'm not so sure about that either."

You see, my performance in the other sections was stellar, and this huge discrepancy could potentially be seen as nothing other than a fluke. But maybe not. "Let me think about it," she said, before walking me to the door of her office and wishing me a fun weekend.

In hindsight, my study strategy certainly had some pitfalls. The MCAT is not about the material itself, but rather about your ability to integrate what you know with the information in the passage in order to answer a question in an average of less than 68 seconds. By the third question of my test, I realized that I had gone about studying for the test completely incorrectly. "Aldosterone is a steroid hormone produced by the adrenal cortex," read the first line of the passage. "I know that," I remember internally congratulating myself. I then went on to read another three paragraphs of information that I did not know, and would not have studied even if I had been given myself a year of prep time. The passage told me everything that I needed to know to answer the questions, and I had wasted time trying to anticipate what information would be necessary to know and trying to memorize those facts. I realized in that second that knowing this information was not the point. The time I had spent learning this and similar facts was time that would have been better spent tackling practice questions, identifying the types of questions that I was getting wrong, and developing strategies to improve those problem areas. It was clear that this had been an issue in my study plan.

About a week later, after my pre-med advisor had conferred with the rest of the advisors in her office, her email read something like this: "After speaking with several of my colleagues, we all agreed that the distribution of your scores is unlike anything we have seen in the short time since the new test has been in circulation. We worry that a better score overall would be hard to achieve, and would certainly hate to see that number drop should you decide to take the test again. However, we are concerned about your low performance on the Bio/Biochem section of the exam, and worry that an admissions committee would see you as a risky candidate and would ultimately lean to rejecting your application. The final decision will be based on which outcome you are more comfortable with."

Huh?

So I could take the test again, but only if I made sure that my overall score wouldn't drop. I could also *not* take the test again, and hope that admissions committees would see this as a fluke. If I took the test and my score dropped, it would probably look like my first, high score was a fluke, and all that time spent studying would have been for nothing. But, if I took the test again and managed to increase my biology score without dropping my overall score, my MCAT could be a glowing piece of my application.

Is your head spinning? Mine sure was.

I thought I had done well the first time. I had studied and prepared the best way I knew how. How could I be sure that my second attempt would be more successful? Where would

I find the time for a full-blown two months of studying before my application was due? Would it be worth delaying my application for another year to bring this score up? How much does it actually matter that one of my scores was low if all the other numbers were within the average for my schools of choice? Would this be *the* thing that kept me off interview guest lists?

The thought of having to retake the MCAT was devastating for several reasons. First, there remains this consistent confusion around what is appropriate; what will look good, bad, or fishy to a medical school admissions committee; where losses should be cut; where excuses should be made; where "good enough" should be accepted. The threshold at which performance on a particular piece of your application becomes poor enough that it is worth the time and effort required to recreate it is fuzzy at best. In fact, looking back, I think it was the process of having to make this decision, rather than the preparation for the second test itself, that became the greatest stressor in my medical school application process.

Second, the MCAT requires a significant time commitment that I did not want to dedicate. Delaying my MCAT would have meant delaying my application for another year, and committing myself to a second gap year, during which time I would not be preparing to pursue medicine.

Here is what actually happened.

Late January, after endless conversations with family, peers, and mentors that were either medical students or graduates,

I finally committed to re-sitting for the MCAT. I knew, as has been told to all pre-med students since Day 1, that your chances of a successful application cycle are highest if you apply at the beginning of the cycle, as admissions decisions are made on a rolling basis. The beginning of the cycle is in early June. I was not willing to spend the time and effort required to apply to medical school without being able to put my best foot forward, so I knew the latest date I could sit for the test and still apply for entry in the cycle that I wanted would be late May. In the six months that stood between me and my proposed test date, I would have to finish up my last semester of undergraduate classes, while, of course, working to maintain my GPA, spending time with my friends, and relishing in the final moments of my undergraduate career, all the while studying and sitting for an exam on which I had already given my best attempt. The sheer timing would make this endeavor nearly impossible.

Another option would be to push the test date and take the MCAT at the end of the summer after graduation. As I mentioned, this would have meant delaying my application another year. This is an option that, in hindsight, I wish I had given more thought. Whether a two-month delay in my application submission would have been *the* only thing to keep me off of acceptance lists is doubtful, but, if you can see a theme emerging here, I was bending over backward to keep these *things* to an absolute minimum.

The thought of delaying my application another year was where the stress levels peaked. Because of the way medical school, residency, and fellowship is chronologically designed, it is not uncommon to hear medical school hopefuls speaking about their lives in five- or ten-year chunks. I was no different.

Delaying my application by a year meant that, assuming there was no significant decrease between my first and second score and that I was actually accepted to medical school the first time I applied, I would be 24 at the time I started. I would be 28 when I finished, and would complete a residency between the ages of 31 and 33 and a fellowship likely by my late 30s. At that point I would have the time, energy, and financial security to have children, a house, a real, grown-up life. All of this already seemed to be eons into the future, and I was not willing to delay it any more than I had to.

Because I am, perhaps, too optimistic at times, I decided to sit for the test again, convincing myself that if I did not get into my dream schools, I would spend the rest of my life wondering whether it was that score that did it. I also made the questionable decision to *not* put my best foot forward and register for a test date that would keep me on track for submitting my full application, but would not give me the time I would need to properly prepare.

In case I haven't mentioned it already, I have come to the realization, now almost two full years after completing my entire written application process, that there is not *one* thing that stands between you and your dream school.

But back to the re-sit. I was underprepared and left the exam unhappy with my performance. As I sat for the last five minutes of my test, all of the conflicting advice I had gotten about the exam throughout my last four years as a pre-med student rushed through my head. *"Don't cancel the score—you definitely performed better than you think you did!"* *"If you are not happy with what you did, cancel and give yourself another shot!"* And then my own concerns: *When would I be able to take it again? There is no third shot. I really just want to be done with this s**t.* All I needed was a set of numbers that would prove to an admissions committee that I could handle the pressures and fast pace of a medical education, and that I could become the doctor I knew I had in me. The first score was not good enough to prove that; maybe the second one would be. I didn't cancel the score. I pressed the button, left the exam room, and drove to a Godiva store to drown my sorrows in a box of caramel truffles.

Of my second set of numbers, three out of four sections, including the Bio/Biochem section I had worked so hard to improve, were exactly the same as my first, down to the percentile ranking. The Psych/Soc section in which I had been most successful on my first attempt had dropped precipitously, bringing down my overall score. I was sure this validated the concerns of any admissions officer who would doubt my ability to perform on standardized tests. To say I was devastated would be an understatement—not even chocolate was doing the trick.

I cried, I yelled, I upgraded to ice cream. I also briefly considered testing for a *third* time, and called every school on my target list to ask their admissions officers how they would view that choice. While I absolutely recommend calling your target schools to have conversations with real humans, I should say that about 90% of these conversations were not that useful. After laying out my two sets of scores, my GPA, and my intent to apply to each admissions officer that I spoke to, I got a lot of answers, such as "It really will depend on the rest of your application," or "We will take both scores into consideration—don't worry," or the absolutely *fantastic* "When thinking about taking the MCAT a third time, you really should look to yourself and ask if that is something you want to do." Okay, obviously I don't *want* to do it, I am asking if it will help me get into your med school, lady.

Finally (and I do mean finally, because I got this response from school 17 of 18 on my list), I spoke with the Dean of Admissions at one of my favorite medical schools, who spoke with me for 20 minutes by phone and explained *how* I should approach this decision. Here are the highlights of that conversation:

- It is statistically impossible to "accidentally" do well on the MCAT. It is, however, possible to have a bad day and to perform poorly. While all schools will consider your scores differently, I [and he said this] imagine that every admissions officer in this country knows that a good MCAT score is more telling of your abilities than a poor one is.

- While we do want to be understanding of poor performance, especially for applicants who otherwise present very strongly, there is only so much justifying that we can do on our end for any given student.

- No one will even blink at a second MCAT score—it happens. And if you really do need to take a third one in order to be competitive at schools you would be happy attending, fine. But, if you do take the MCAT a third time, you need to treat preparation for that exam like preparation for an Olympic sport.

Fast-forward seven months and I am sitting in my first interview. The woman sitting on the other side of the desk concluded a wonderful, 45-minute chat with *"Last question, Elisabeth, and I really have to ask. Why did you take the MCAT again?"* My expression must have given away my feeling about this *horrible* decision, because she started chuckling. I think I pieced together a coherent response to the tune of "I didn't feel like my score in the Biology section reflected my understanding of those topics…," but even as I muttered this partial truth, I began to realize a couple of important things that are a bit more explanatory.

First, why I really retook the MCAT was a combination of fear and hope: fear that this score would be that *one* thing, that one wrong decision that would keep me off interview invitation lists, and hope that I had not just spent three years of my life and hundreds of thousands of dollars studying Molecular and Cellular Biology at an elite university to come out only partially knowing biology, and that AMCAS had made some kind of mistake when they released my scores.

Second, I truly did know that my performance would be poor the second time I took the test, even as I pulled up woefully unprepared, coffee in hand, to the strip mall where I would take my test. "Let's just get this over with," I thought to myself, and I truly meant it. I was so excited to rid myself of the weight of this test that I completely lost sight of why I was there at all. By this point, the MCAT had been on my radar for almost a year. When I wasn't studying for it, I was planning a prep schedule, waiting for scores to come out, and weighing in my head the importance of my scores in determining my future career. This entire process had emotionally and physically exhausted me. Had I pushed through this short-term distress, I would have likely come out with a better result, worthy of the effort required for a re-sit. Retaking the exam is never ideal, and a decision that should be made with meticulous certainty, commitment, and zeal. However, it should also be made within a reasonable time frame—more than anything in this process, the preparation leading up to the MCAT is a marathon, not a sprint.

Third, I recognize that the very thought of cancelling a score after spending countless hours studying and actually sitting through more than seven hours of testing feels like you are cutting off your own foot—or at least, it did to me. The decision actually seemed so extreme that even though I had spent the entire test physically uncomfortable—the room was cold, I had a cold, and my mouse trackpad was not functioning properly—I brushed the idea aside almost as a nonstarter before I had even sat down. What's more, the experience did not get any better as the day went on. In the Chem/Phys section, I found myself stuck on one math problem for more than three minutes, an absolute no-no in the world of testing. In the Psych/Soc section, which had been my highest score on my first test, I found myself clicking through answers almost entirely by chance, burned out by the last section of the test both from the testing itself and from the weeks I had spent studying. Yes, I did have some hope that my concerns were unfounded or exaggerated, but I was so desperate to rid myself of the MCAT entirely that the decision to keep my scores was one made from desperation, rather than from confidence.

Finally, any decision to re-sit should be based on a fundamental understanding of what could have been done differently, and a near certainty that any changes in attitude, study strategy, or pure knowledge attainment will make a difference in your score. I realized after the fact that I had not made very fruitful changes in my study habits. Sure, I had done more practice tests and focused less on memorizing material, but I had also changed aspects of my study habits that I have known to be successful for years. What I was left with was a haphazard attempt to master material using strategies I was neither familiar with nor committed to. I had never been more unprepared for an exam than I had been on that day, and it showed.

So the moral of this narrative is that this one score was not worth the time, money, or commitment that I needed to dedicate in order to see marked improvements. I took the MCAT in my Senior spring and missed a lot of enjoyable college experiences because I chose to devote my time to studying. Even then, I was not particularly thrilled about my decision to sit again, so my studying was not as productive or strategically planned as a test like this demands. I was also in classes at the time, and I was not able to study the way that I knew was most successful for me. Instead of listening to my gut, I attempted to plow my way through it in less-than-ideal conditions for the sake of getting it done. I was left annoyed at the experiences I was missing out on and disillusioned as all the hours I was committing felt as if they were getting me nowhere.

ACTIVITIES LIST | 6

Remember that fabulously diverse group of advisors we interviewed while working on this book? The ones that let me in on the little-known secrets of the medical school admissions process? Well, they also spoke to me about the list of experiences and activities that a student will need to craft a competitive application, and got me thinking about how to craft this list for acceptance.

Let's get something out of the way here: if adcoms are asking you to include it in the application, then they are committing themselves to read it—for you, and for the 5,000+ other applicants who will be crossing their desks every single season. If they are making a commitment like that, the information they are asking you to provide here must be very important to their assessment process. Don't waste their time by giving them information of little value.

The purpose of the activities list and the descriptive blurbs is to help adcoms determine whether:

1. You possess the soft skills that will make you a good doctor.

2. You have amassed enough exposure to the field of medicine to know (rather than just think you know) that you want to be a doctor.

3. Their graduating class will be made up of students with a wealth of diverse experiences.

I know what you're thinking: I just spent the last 50 pages of this book convincing you that the GPA and MCAT scores are the two most important pieces of the application. So then, what gives? Isn't keeping a competitive GPA, spending months studying for the MCAT, trying to graduate from college on time, and attempting to pay for college all enough to prove that you can handle the emotional and physical stress of medical school and then medical practice?

Well, you would think. But no.

Once they've established which students can handle the academic rigor of medical school, adcoms will be on the lookout for those special applicants who possess the soft skills required to be successful physician. This includes cultural competency, teamwork, oral and written communication skills, perseverance, grit, ability to deal with ambiguity, curiosity about the world around you, and the ability to relate to people.

The AAMC* has actually published a list of 15 Core Competencies, ratified by medical schools across the country, that highlight what these most important soft skills are:

INTERPERSONAL COMPETENCIES	
Service Orientation	Demonstrates a desire to help others and sensitivity to others' needs and feelings; demonstrates a desire to alleviate others' distress; recognizes and acts on his/her responsibilities to society; locally, nationally, and globally.
Social Skills	Demonstrates an awareness of others' needs, goals, feelings, and the ways that social and behavioral cues affect peoples' interactions and behaviors; adjusts behaviors appropriately in response to these cues; treats others with respect.
Cultural Competence	Demonstrates knowledge of socio-cultural factors that affect interactions and behaviors; shows an appreciation and respect for multiple dimensions of diversity; recognizes and acts on the obligation to inform one's own judgment; engages diverse and competing perspectives as a resource for learning, citizenship, and work; recognizes and appropriately addresses bias in themselves and others; interacts effectively with people from diverse backgrounds.
Teamwork	Works collaboratively with others to achieve shared goals; shares information and knowledge with others and provides feedback; puts team goals ahead of individual goals.
Oral Communication	Effectively conveys information to others using spoken words and sentences; listens effectively; recognizes potential communication barriers and adjusts approach or clarifies information as needed.

INTRAPERSONAL COMPETENCIES	
Ethical Responsibility to Self and Others	Behaves in an honest and ethical manner; cultivates personal and academic integrity; adheres to ethical principles and follows rules and procedures; resists peer pressure to engage in unethical behavior and encourages others to behave in honest and ethical ways; develops and demonstrates ethical and moral reasoning.
Reliability and Dependability	Consistently fulfills obligations in a timely and satisfactory manner; takes responsibility for personal actions and performance.
Resilience and Adaptability	Demonstrates tolerance of stressful or changing environments or situations and adapts effectively to them; is persistent, even under difficult situations; recovers from setbacks.
Capacity for Improvement	Sets goals for continuous improvement and for learning new concepts and skills; engages in reflective practice for improvement; solicits and responds appropriately to feedback.

THINKING AND REASONING COMPETENCIES	
Critical Thinking	Uses logic and reasoning to identify the strengths and weaknesses of alternative solutions, conclusions, or approaches to problems.
Quantitative Reasoning	Applies quantitative reasoning and appropriate mathematics to describe or explain phenomena in the natural world.
Scientific Inquiry	Applies knowledge of the scientific process to integrate and synthesize information, solve problems and formulate research questions and hypotheses; is facile in the language of the sciences and uses it to participate in the discourse of science and explain how scientific knowledge is discovered and validated.
Written Communication	Effectively conveys information to others using written words and sentences.
SCIENCE COMPETENCIES	
Living Systems	Applies knowledge and skill in the natural sciences to solve problems related to molecular and macro systems including biomolecules, molecules, cells, and organs.
Human Behavior	Applies knowledge of the self, others, and social systems to solve problems related to the psychological, socio-cultural, and biological factors that influence health and well-being.

In summary, this stuff is pretty darn important.

So then what does this have to do with the activities list? Well, unfortunately, there won't be an option to just tell the schools you possess these coveted doctor-like traits.

If you possess soft skills, check here: ☐

What you will have is the opportunity to fill in 15 slots with activities, experiences, or awards, and will be given 700 characters to write about **what you did, what you learned, and how it impacted your personal journey to medical school.** "I worked in a lab" is NOT a description. Each of your 700-character blurbs MUST encompass WHAT you did, WHAT you learned, and HOW it impacted your personal journey to medical school.

For the three experiences that you designate as "most meaningful experiences" you will get an extra 1,325 characters to let adcoms know why that is. Again, keep those important details in mind as you write.

All of your experiences will fall broadly into one of the following categories—or, they should, because these are the categories in the drop-down menu on AMCAS that you will get to choose from when you are describing them:

1. Paid employment—not medical/clinical

2. Paid employment—medical/clinical

3. Teaching/Tutoring/Teaching assistant

4. Research/Lab

5. Community Service/Volunteer—medical/clinical

6. Community Service/Volunteer—not medical/clinical

7. Physician shadowing/clinical observation

8. Honors/awards/recognitions

9. Artistic endeavors

10. Extracurricular activities

11. Leadership—not listed elsewhere

12. Other

Now why would I take up space to list these categories for you when you could just find them online? Because we can glean from them some very important insight into the minds of the medical school admissions officers—namely, what they value in their applicants and what experiences they consider to be particularly important!

Myth: You definitely have to have research, shadowing, and clinical volunteering experience to get into medical school.

I'm sure you have heard this advice multiple times from your friends, pre-professional advisors, Reddit, or elsewhere about how to get into medical school. And don't get me wrong—it makes sense. I mean, after all, these are the most doctor-y things on that list, and I definitely recommend hitting these categories in some way before submitting your application. However, as with everything in life, there are caveats to how you should pursue each one. There is a lot of potential value in pursuing activities within the other nonmedical categories on that list as well—so much so that you would probably be at a disadvantage if you tried to artificially limit yourself to these Big Three.

The point is that we recognize *why* each of these categories could be important and *how* they might suggest to an adcom that you have the values and skills they are looking for in their future physicians. Being able to pull out those themes will help guide you in your writing and allow you to produce the best and most valuable "descriptions" to go along with your title and category. Let's walk through each category and try to figure out a potential value add.

PAID EMPLOYMENT—MEDICAL/ CLINICAL OR NOT

Medical schools want to attract a diverse group of students to their incoming class, and while "diversity" can seem at times like an overused buzzword, it definitely holds a lot of value to adcoms. Paid employment could very well signify to a committee that you can add some of the economic diversity they seek. Medical/clinical paid employment is ideal if you can find it, but adcoms will not hold it against you if you have fewer experiences across the other categories, or less medical-related experience overall, because you were working to support yourself.

Teaching/Tutoring/Teaching Assistant

WHY DO THEY WANT TO SEE IT?

As a doctor, you will be charged with teaching your patients and inspiring them to take charge of their own health. If you can't do that, you are a technician, not a physician, and that is exactly how admissions committees will look at you if you do not have at least *something* in this category.

HOW CAN YOU FIND EXPERIENCES TO FILL THIS CATEGORY?

This category could be fulfilled doing literally any type of teaching. Do you coach a soccer team? Tutor kids in a foreign language? TA for your General Chemistry class? Anything and everything can be entered here.

A STRONG DESCRIPTION IN THIS CATEGORY:

The grammar and syntax I teach in my first grade classroom are challenging. The rules often have no obvious reason for implementation and each explanation is specific to the verb or noun group we are working on. Each question posed by a student is an opportunity. To address an inquiry in a clear, timely, and comprehensible manner requires consistent focus and decisiveness on my part. I am confident that the capacity to remain calm and collected while teaching will serve me well as my work shifts from the classroom to a hospital. The patience needed to teach patients about their health was born in that first grade classroom.

A NOT-SO-STRONG DESCRIPTION IN THIS CATEGORY:

I have taught grammar to first graders while volunteering as a weekend aid in an underserved area near my university.

RESEARCH/LAB

WHY DO THEY WANT TO SEE IT?

Throughout your career as a physician, you will be (largely) responsible for keeping up with your continued education. You will do this mostly by reading up on the latest published articles on the effects of pharmaceuticals and medical procedures for your particular patient population. Having a frame of reference for *how* that research was produced will make you a better consumer of information, and, therefore, a more informed and helpful doctor. And before you ask, no—you do not have to get published to put it on your application!

HOW CAN YOU FIND EXPERIENCES TO FILL THIS CATEGORY?

There are two ways to go about this:

1. **Determine a topic that interests you and then find a place to do your research.** This will be easiest for those of you that are studying at or live near large research universities. If that is the case for you, dedicate some time figuring out what interests you. I recommend starting out easy, such as looking at the "health" section of your favorite online newspaper or magazine to see what research is being talked about.

Once you get a sense of what is out there in lay terms, delve into academic articles. See what you understand and what sparks your interest. Remember, you will likely be dedicating a lot of time and effort into a very focused piece of research, so it better be something that excites you, or the hours you spend in the lab will be absolutely miserable. When you have located a topic, look at which professors on your campus or in your city are dedicated to that work.

2. **Find whatever work you can and make yourself interested in what is available.** Although this method is less than ideal, it may be the best option for you if you live in a medically underserved community or don't have access to a lot of research-producing institutions. Even if it is not your favorite topic in the world, the benefits you will gain from designing and executing experiments will undoubtedly give you a leg up on your application journey, and may be worth at least a *bit* of your time to gain that exposure.

A STRONG DESCRIPTION IN THIS CATEGORY

Under the guidance and leadership of Dr. X, I worked with senior scientists studying the immunological mechanisms of disease Y. I assisted in conducting a comprehensive analysis on the effects of co-signaling molecules on T-cell expression by employing PCRs, Western blots, SDS-gels, and computational analysis of flow cytometry data. Dr. X and his team were gracious enough to teach me all of these techniques. This experience was my first exposure to the practical implications of the science I was learning in the classroom. As a result, it allowed me insight into the life and work of a physician-scientist and ignited my passion for medicine.

A NOT-SO-STRONG DESCRIPTION IN THIS CATEGORY

While in college, I worked in a lab studying the effects of X on Disease Y. While I did not publish a paper, I felt I learned a lot from this experience, and would like to continue work like this throughout medical school.

COMMUNITY SERVICE/VOLUNTEER— MEDICAL/CLINICAL AND NOT

WHY DO THEY WANT TO SEE IT?

So much of your career as a doctor will be dependent on helping people, and "I want to help people" is a fairly common answer to the age-old question "Why do you want to be a doctor?" While that is easy to say, it does require some kind of commitment to show. It's hard to convince an admissions committee that you want to commit your life to the service of others without having spent any time doing that throughout your pre-med years.

HOW CAN YOU FIND EXPERIENCES TO FILL THIS CATEGORY?

Volunteer work need not be exclusively medical or clinical. In fact, some of the most unique and rewarding experiences will come from you dedicating your time and your gifts to the betterment of your community. If you like to cook, teach a cooking class at a rec center. If you like to play the piano, spend a few hours a week playing in a retirement community. I like to sing, so I would organize my collegiate *a cappella* group once every few months to put on a show for the children's neuromuscular unit in the hospital near our college campus. The goal here is to highlight your character. Are you willing to give of yourself to others without being asked?

In addition to turning your nonmedical passions into volunteer opportunities, medical or clinical volunteer work can also be deeply rewarding, with the added bonus of giving you exposure to the environment in which you aim to spend your career. Whichever way you ultimately decide to do this, use these experiences to hone in on what makes you tick. Try to describe what it is about offering your services to others that will distinguish your "I like to help people" personal statement or interview response from the thousands of others like it.

A STRONG DESCRIPTION IN THIS CATEGORY

Volunteering at Children's Hospital solidified my desire to become a physician. I had the opportunity to witness the impact of the doctors, who served not only as caretakers for patients, but as confidants and cheerleaders for their parents as well. The physicians who were best able to inspire confidence, calm, and trust in their patients' parents were those most in touch with the problems that accompanied the illness of their child. Whether involving the logistics of splitting time with another, healthy child, or concerns

> about scheduling and finances, parents held the
> weight of an entire life outside the hospital walls. The
> best doctors were adept at shouldering some of this
> burden.

A NOT-SO-STRONG DESCRIPTION IN THIS CATEGORY

> I have spent 280 hours volunteering at Children's
> Hospital. My responsibilities on my weekly three-
> hour shifts included playing with the kids, keeping
> them occupied, and cleaning up after them.

PHYSICIAN SHADOWING/CLINICAL OBSERVATION

WHY DO THEY WANT TO SEE IT?

Despite all the hype about getting an acceptance to medical school, the time you will spend there is just a detour on the way to the ultimate goal: the practice of medicine. In addition to being confident that you can get through their curriculum and pass the national licensure exam to actually be able to practice medicine, medical schools also want to know that all the time and energy they are going to put into making you a doctor will not go to waste. That means that they have to be convinced that you know and possess what it takes to practice medicine. They need to know that you are aware of what you're getting yourself into. Now obviously you won't know *exactly* what it's like until you get the opportunity to actually do it, but you can speak more persuasively and with greater confidence about your excitement to be a doctor if you have at least a bit of exposure.

HOW CAN YOU FIND EXPERIENCES TO FILL THIS CATEGORY?

Getting shadowing or clinical experience will be highly dependent on how comfortable you are reaching out to people. If you have any family members or friends of your parents who are doctors, reach out to them first. You can also try your own doctor. If you want to know about a particular type of medicine, look at hospitals or private practices in your area and reach out to people via their online profiles or office phone numbers. You would be surprised what a positive response you can get from just an enthusiastic cold call.

Separate from the admissions game, gaining exposure to different specialties and types of medical practice will help you get a sense of how you would like to join the field. It will also give you a better idea of what to aim for in your future practice—after all, the day in the life of an urban private-practice cardiologist is a lot different from the life of a general practitioner in a rural hospital, and you won't know what is best for you until you give each a try. Get as much exposure as you can here. If you do have parents who are doctors, definitely take the opportunity to shadow them, but try to get some *additional experience as well*. Not only will a lot of different exposure be an impressive addition to your application, but you also don't want to give admissions committees the impression that you were not committed enough to reach out past your immediate circle.

A STRONG DESCRIPTION IN THIS CATEGORY

I had the opportunity to observe firsthand the work environment, pace, and responsibilities of a hematologist, while also being privy to Dr. X's interactions with her patients. She was able to put patients at ease with her calm and professional demeanor. Admirably, she maintained this demeanor in the face of presenting life-altering news or test results, despite the unique challenges presented by each individual patient. The empathy, knowledge, and decisiveness she exhibited gave me the example of excellence that I hope to emulate in my own career.

A NOT-SO-STRONG DESCRIPTION IN THIS CATEGORY

I have spent 130 hours shadowing Dr. X on her oncology rounds and watching her interact with patients.

Why Activities Matter

We will now be shifting gears into the next goal of activities. While the activity categories above serve to persuade admissions committees that you have what it takes to become a good doctor, the remaining activity categories, namely honors/awards/recognitions, artistic endeavors, extracurricular activities, leadership and other, serve a dual purpose. These give you space and opportunity to highlight the experiences that helped shape you into a strong candidate and allow medical school admissions committees to meet that part of you. Ideally, you will have something to say about each of the categories described in detail above, with the exception, perhaps, of paid work. However, collecting experiences across nonmedical categories will more likely give you fodder to write a compelling personal statement or to provide interesting anecdotes than it will be to convince the admissions committee that you would make a good physician.

While most schools are fairly flexible with their requirements on the activities front, some may be particular about you having accumulated certain types of experiences. The most common examples are schools that require clinical experience or to complete a set number of volunteer hours. I know it's hard to know exactly what schools you will be applying to until you get to that point, but even having a tentative list will help you avoid any unwanted "I-don't-have-enough-service-hours-to-apply-to-my-dream-school-this-cycle" type surprises.

So how important is this list?

A close priority #2 after GPA and MCAT. To quote a former admissions officer who was kind enough to speak to me about this book,

> **"Lack of experience is the #1 reason** that applicants with otherwise excellent applications don't get into medical school."

It is also the #2 area of improvement (after an increased MCAT score) that admissions officers look for when assessing re-applicants for admission.

How should you go about creating this list?

Think about what qualities *you* think an excellent doctor embodies and how those fit in with the med-school-ratified AAMC Core Competencies. These are the traits that you should build your activities list and associated descriptions around, with whatever experiences spark your interest and highlight your passions.

Just remember, adcoms have heard it all, so you likely won't impress them by coming up with the coolest-activity-there-ever-was and dedicating your time to that. Instead, *you will impress them with your commitment, leadership, and impact within an experience that thousands of students before you have participated in.* So, as you try to figure out how to spend your time, think about the following:

1. **Am I enjoying this activity?** Do I go there with excitement about the time I will spend, or am I counting down the minutes before my time even starts?

2. **What am I getting out of this activity?** If your answer to this question is "A glitzy line item on my application," then I would run—not walk—in the opposite direction.

3. **How does this activity relate to my passion for medicine?** This is not to say that it has to be directly related to the medical field, but rather that it should highlight he same qualities you aim to embody as a physician.

WHAT SHOULD YOU DO AS YOU PARTICIPATE?

Keep a journal as you go to track the benefits you receive and the impacts you make (it will be easier to write when the time comes), and you should be all set by the time you need to fill out this part of the application.

WRITING THE
PERSONAL STATEMENT | 7

Your personal statement is the first opportunity you will
have to show adcoms who you are and what key moments,
people, and events have led you to submit this application.
It is where you get to weave together the experiences,
activities, thoughts, and personal growth that has taken
place throughout your life (with special emphasis given
to your pre-med years, of course), into a poignant, clear,
and well-written essay about why you want to be a doctor.
Oh, and you get to do it all in under 5,300 characters
if you are submitting the AMCAS, 4,500 characters if
you're submitting the AACOMAS, or 5,000 characters if
you're submitting the TMDSAS. If you're submitting the
TMDSAS, you will also get up to 5,000 additional characters
across a "personal characteristics essay" (2,500 characters)
and an optional essay (2,500 characters), which is an
"opportunity to provide the admissions committee(s) with
a broader picture of who you are as an applicant." If you
are lucky enough to be submitting primary applications to
more than one of these applications, you will get to tweak
your main "Why do you want to be a doctor" essay to fit the
specifications of each.

Your essay is meant to answer the ultimate question of why
you want to be a doctor. You will talk about experiences

you've had to prove that you know what you're talking about, and about personal revelations that have brought you to medicine. You should start drafting this essay as soon as possible, and thinking about what resources you have available that can help improve your essay. My recommendation would be to start drafting as early as December before the application opens.

For all of you procrastinators out there who just rolled your eyes at that, do consider it. It is harder than it seems to write in a way that is compelling but not overly descriptive, that portrays your compassion without sounding naïve or condescending, and that highlights your contribution without sounding self-righteous. All these nuances, by the way, will likely require input from someone else (may even multiple others), and I can almost guarantee all these people won't be able to turn it around as fast you need it if you try to start on May 26.

Finally, probably the most important thing to remember about writing a personal statement: *you are not going to tell any adcoms anything they haven't already heard.* Don't waste your time racking your brain in an attempt to stand out from the crowd because of *content.* Try instead to sift through your experiences to find the ones you can write about in the most compelling way. The "sell" here is how the experience impacted you and how it has changed your goals, passions, and course of action.

Now I know some of you are thinking that while most people write certain variations of a few similar themes, *your* essay is definitely different. It will be unique and special because you are unique and special, and this uniqueness is why adcoms will fall in love with you. I really hope that is the case for you. But in case it isn't, let's get these common essay topics out in the open and talk about how you *can* distinguish yourself from, well, everyone else that is thinking the same thing.

The Personal Statement is intended to give you some space where you can write about *why* you want to be a doctor. The topic itself is a bit leading, so it's no wonder so many applicants are led in one of these directions:

I want to be a doctor because…

1. I really like to help people.

2. I am passionate about science and want to apply it in a tangible way.

3. I have excellent people skills, and would enjoy a career working with others.

4. My parents are doctors.

5. Doctors enjoy a lot of money and/or prestige.

What NOT to Write

Let's get something out in the open from the beginning: If you are planning on writing about #4 or #5, let me save you the application fees now. It won't work. In fact, it will do the opposite of getting you in. It will fill the heads of your committee members with doubts about your intentions and about your ability to thrive in the medical field without really feeling that medicine is your calling. This is an important point. When I was an undergrad, I went to an admissions event for a selective medical school in Massachusetts where the school's director of admissions spoke. Expecting to hear the same things I had heard from every other similar event I had attended (e.g., our school has great research and a wonderful community, apply to us even if you think you won't get in, blah blah blah), he started his piece in a way that really stuck with me. He told an auditorium full of excited, exhausted, and nervous upperclassmen that medicine is one of the *worst* careers in the world. The pay per hour is horrible, the quality of life is dictated by on-call schedules, and your required commitment to your patients makes it essentially a service job.

I would argue that it is actually the world's *ultimate* service job because you actually have very little flexibility or choice about responding to your patients' needs. You can't ignore them in the hope that they will get the hint and change their bad behavior; you can't power through with dreams of a commission on the other side; you can't even refuse to take them on as a client. That patient becomes a part of your life the second their health is in your hands. Thus, your commitment to them is extraordinary.

So then even if medicine is a particularly grueling *job,* this admissions officer continued, it is an outstanding *calling.* Those who go into medicine do so because they are called to serve others in a way that very few have the privilege to.

You will get to deliver children and treat cancers, to calm your patients' nerves and to teach them to take better care of their minds and bodies. Your adcoms likely know better than you do what a privilege it is to have the opportunity to attend medical school and get the skills necessary to serve your community in that particular way. While they know that you can't possibly fathom the weight of that privilege just yet, they want to *at least* see that you've tried.

If you are going into medicine for the money, sorry to break it to you, but that is definitely not a smart move. Yes, doctors make an excellent living, and yes, I'm sure that is a perk to which every pre-med and medical student is looking forward. However, there are many, *many* hurdles to cross before you get there and even more ways to get rich faster and easier than through a medical degree. If money is your goal, I would recommend going into finance or technology, or trying your luck at the lottery.

Similarly, telling an admissions committee that you want to attend their medical school because your parents are doctors just screams "I DON'T KNOW WHAT ELSE TO DO WITH MY LIFE so let me in please, K?"

Again, not a great impression to leave on an adcom. Even if you think you have a perfect way of weaving it into your story of how they inspired you to pursue this path, don't do it. Just don't even type out the words. Plus, they will know that your parents are doctors based on the parental information and will probably assume that it has had some impact on your decision.

The *only* exception is if you shadowed your parents/relatives and had an experience with a patient that made you want to pursue medicine. Noble? Absolutely. However, even then, I would tread cautiously. It is very hard to write "around" the fact that you were exposed to this opportunity because of your parents, and even harder to get out of the reader's head that deep down inside, that relationship may be influencing your application. My recommendation? I'm sure your doctor-relative has some other doctor-friends, right? Shadow them instead and steer clear of this whole debacle.

If you were planning on making either of these reasons the centerpiece of your personal statement, or even worse, if either of these points actually is the reason you want to go into medicine, then do yourself a favor—find a more suitable career.

What to Write

As far as the first three common themes: "I want to be a doctor so I can help people," "I like science," and "I like working with people." These are all *fine* reasons to want to become a doctor. However, if you have picked any of these to write about and that is *all* you plan on saying, you are setting yourself up to produce a lackluster piece of writing. They won't hold up in a competitive pool if they are on their own, so you will definitely have to go the extra mile with all of these.

For example, there are plenty of careers that allow you to help people, both inside (nurse, physical therapist, occupational therapist, etc.) and outside (air traffic controller, teacher) of the healthcare field. *A good essay* will note that doctors help people, so you can write about how attractive that makes medicine to you. However, a great essay will call out what differentiates (in your eyes) a doctor from all the other people-helping careers that are out there.

The same logic applies to theme #3. Yes, a desire to work with people will be instrumental as you progress in the medical field, but certainly not sufficient to highlight your commitment to the practice of medicine to an adcom. You'll have to go further than that. What is special about the doctor-patient relationship in particular that it is different from the patient's relationship with their nurse, occupational therapist, teacher, waitress, lawyer, or realtor?

Not to freak you out—I am fairly certain that you will not be asked why you prefer serving patients over selling houses at any point in your admissions process. However, the idea still stands: if your essay leaves the committee with even a sliver of doubt as to your commitment to this particular profession, with all of its challenges, nuances, and obstacles, then chances are they won't want to speak to you in person.

Finally, you can state "I am good at" (or even better—"I really like") "biology, chemistry, anatomy, physiology, etc." as a good way to answer the "why do you want to be a doctor" question and address a skillset that will serve you well as you continue in the medical profession. But if this is all you say, you will have missed a golden opportunity to craft a *great* essay by linking skills in these areas to the service of your community.

Again, a mediocre personal statement is not a reason to reject you. But it certainly won't be a reason to accept you either, and the way the numbers in this process work, each interviewee and accepted student has demonstrated that there is a reason to accept them. The personal statement is 5,300-ish characters worth of opportunity for you to give them that reason.

Common Pitfalls to Avoid

The most common mistake I've seen from students is personal statements that are completely descriptive—almost like a timeline of their pre-medical careers. They go for breadth instead of depth, and end up with a laundry list of haphazardly described experiences that fall short of making a compelling narrative. The Personal Statement is the one piece of writing you can use to describe your passion and enthusiasm for this profession that has you spending your undergraduate years in ultra-challenging courses, your weekends volunteering in hospital wards, and your summers toiling away at cell cultures in a freezing cold lab. Telling us that you did those things won't be enough (because basically everyone has, and because that's what your activities list is for). What you have to let shine through in your writing is *why* you did it, and why it was exciting and interesting for you.

That excitement is what will set you apart from other applicants who spend too much time focusing on what they did instead of *why* they did it. The trick is finding a way to channel the passion and enthusiasm that has seen you through years of preparing to write this essay into an honest, persuasive, and authentic recounting of what made you want to dedicate your life to the practice of medicine. Remember when I told you to start the January before applications open?

In order to craft a personal statement, here are some handy techniques and questions to get you thinking.

WHAT TRAITS AND VALUES DO YOU ENVISION BRINGING TO YOUR PRACTICE OF MEDICINE?

You may not know yet what specialty you want to pursue (which is completely acceptable, because that is bound to change before you graduate anyway), but I bet when you dream of becoming a doctor, you have a vision in your head of exactly what that looks like.

All of the variations on what practicing as a doctor look like are valid, realistic, and have the exact same starting point. As pre-med students, we so often get caught up in focusing on an acceptance letter as the end of the road that we forget it is just the beginning of a long and fruitful journey. Call on those aspirations and visions to persuade an admissions committee that you should get a chance to start.

You may dream of helping the underserved by offering life-saving preventative care in a low-income community. You may dream of conducting clinical trials for fancy cancer drugs. You may even want to be one of the physicians designing those drugs/new technologies. Hopefully, you have been pursuing activities, passions, and interests that honor your vision.

The personal statement is also an opportunity to show your personality and add some flair! But remember to always be appropriate and on topic. Again, this can go right back to what kind of doctor you envision yourself becoming. Do you think a doctor ought to be approachable? Are you approachable? Show the admissions people that the answer is YES by sharing related anecdotes and pulling out poignant "morals" or "lessons learned" from them.

WHAT EXPERIENCE CAN YOU NARRATE THAT CAPTURES WHAT INSPIRED YOU TO START THIS JOURNEY?

Medical school is a long, expensive process. You haven't even begun yet and all of your energy is being dedicated to the pursuit of this career! What's more, the practice of medicine can be exhausting and thankless, and demand more of its practitioners than they are able to give. Assuming you are not some horribly masochistic person who enjoys drowning in student loan debt and anatomy flashcards for the fun of it, there must be some reason deep in the recesses of your mind that has caused you to pursue this particular career path. The Personal Statement is the space dedicated for you to tell that story. If the story has a captivating main character, great! It will certainly help speed your writing process along. If not, you might consider making one up. Human-centered stories give you latitude to be descriptive and should engage the human on the other side of your application.

Even if there isn't a particular moment that turned you on to medicine, think about one that best captures the emotions you feel when you think of yourself with patients of your own one day, and make that the centerpiece of your writing.

WHAT WILL YOU BRING TO YOUR MATRICULATING CLASS?

Be very clear about what makes you unique as an applicant and what diversity (and I mean this in the broadest sense of the word) you will bring to your class. Yes, they are ultimately trying to graduate proficient and ethical doctors, but in order to do so, they will be building a matriculating class whose members they will likely be interacting with during the next four years (adcoms are often made up of school deans, professors, etc.). What that means is your personal statement is an opportunity to not only convince them that should you be a medical student, but also that you should be *their* medical student. This is the opportunity to talk about your emotions, values, and opinions, and why you would be a useful member of the incoming class at Fabulous Medical School. Don't forget, though, this is not the place to get specific about individual medical schools— you will have plenty of opportunities to do that in the secondary application.

"Medicine" is a fairly broad and encompassing term. After medical school, doctors diverge in their pursuits, business models, patient groups, and, of course, specialties. No one is saying that you have to know now what your practice will look like in 10 or 15 years, but you do have to indicate that you have at least thought about it.

I knew that I was passionate about issues of healthcare access and how insurance schemes exclude certain patient populations from accessing care. The problem was that in a very practical sense, I had only "found" this passion about nine months before I originally intended to apply. The depth of my involvement in activities that would give me my view on these issues was lacking. If I wanted healthcare access to be my "thing," I would have to invest time and energy into its development.

For me, that meant pursuing a Master's degree, and later, a job working on health systems design. For you, that might mean spending a year doing volunteer work, taking additional courses, or enhancing your proficiency in a language. Whatever it is, pinpoint it. Start now! The earlier the better, and the more space you give yourself to develop this passion before you submit the application, the better position you will be in! You will want your application centered on a theme that best reflects what particular part of medicine you are passionate about.

To sum up, the personal statement needs to be a well-written, well-thought-out piece of writing that deftly tells the adcoms why you want to be a doctor. It should also show that you have the compassion, drive, grit, and inspiration to get there. Oh, and you should start drafting it… yesterday!

LETTERS OF RECOMMENDATION | 8

The letters of recommendation are the final piece of your primary application, creating another opportunity for you to highlight your strengths and showcase your personality. When you begin the process of requesting letters of recommendation to add to your medical school application, it is important to remember the *who, when, why, and how* of the letter-requesting process.

WHO

Obviously a very important piece of this puzzle is deciding from whom you are going to request letters of recommendation. This is not as straightforward as you think. You are asking someone to the take time to write, uncompensated, in a way that is compelling about your strengths, weaknesses, and growth over the time that they have known you. Ideally, you will have some professors who have a plethora of interactions with you from which to pull when they write.

To get to this point, you want to build relationships with your professors, as soon as you can, in a way that is authentic and organic. There are two really great ways to do this:

1. Get involved in research with your professor.

2. Take advantage of office hours to get to know them in a casual setting.

Getting Involved in Research

Getting involved in research in your professor's lab can be a stellar way to get to know them and to show off your skills in an environment of mutual interest. Of course, that assumes your professor has a lab that accepts undergraduates, that you have the time to commit to research, and, most importantly, that you are actually interested in the research your professor is doing.

This can be accomplished in one of two ways: prioritize the person, or prioritize the work. Either you reach out to a professor that you click with (whose work you also find interesting) for an opportunity to join their lab, or you scope out all the professors in your department and find the one whose work is most interesting to you. Then, make a point of taking a class with that person at some point throughout your studies. The first way is easier, since you are not cold calling someone without any context as to who you are and how useful you could potentially be.

An email for the first scenario could say:

> *Dear Professor SuperCoolResearchProject,*
> *My name is Elisabeth, and I am a Molecular and*
> *Cellular Biology sophomore in your Developmental*
> *Biology class this semester. After learning about topic*
> *X in your lecture this week, I decided to look into this*
> *further and noticed that you are conducting research*
> *on this topic in your lab. I would be thrilled for the*
> *opportunity to work on a project like this if you have*
> *any space available. Would you be around this week*
> *or next to chat about this? Please also find my resume*
> *attached for your reference.*
>
> *Best wishes,*
> *Elisabeth*

Not too bad, right?

On the other hand, the second route, which opens up your reach to any professor on your campus, gives you more flexibility and choices about what to get involved with. The trouble with this is that it may require a lot more persistence on your part. You have no connection to draw with this person, and given the excessive workload that most academics have, your email may not even make it onto their radar. However, if after reading articles on that particular research topic you feel like it is interesting enough that you would be happy dedicating a good chunk of your time to it, be persistent!

Don't be afraid to send follow-up emails or even try to catch the professor in their office if that option is available to you. Go in with the knowledge that undergraduates are helpful and exciting to have around, if only for the fresh enthusiasm they bring to the project. Additionally, these types of gigs rarely pay (or not much anyway), so worst case scenario you are cheap labor, being paid in the opportunity to learn instead of real cash. Never underestimate how valuable that is, especially in the cash-strapped, grant-driven world of academia.

Approaching Professors During Office Hours

Even if you are fortunate enough to get involved in conducting research that interests you with a professor at your undergraduate institution, the one letter from that person will not be enough to cover the "recommendation letter" requirement for medical school. You will also have to engage with your other professors, past and present, in order to get letters of support. This is most likely to happen later in your college career as you progress into smaller, upper-level classes, as opposed to the 300-person, lecture-style courses that will characterize most of freshman and sophomore year. Smaller classes mean more opportunities for professors to interact personally with each student. The added bonus is that smaller classes tend to cover more niche topics specific to the interests (and potentially, academic work) of the professor teaching the course. Since the topics are more interesting for them, they are more likely to want to chat about them. If you get on their good side by discussing topics that interest them, they are more inclined to want to talk to you about your interests as well.

The best way to build a relationship with your professors is to approach them during their scheduled office hours, as this is the time they've carved out to be available for students. I would not recommend "popping in" to try to avoid the crowds, as this can be disruptive and frustrating for professors who undoubtedly have other things on their plate. Rather, try fitting office hours into your schedule as a consistent, weekly occurrence, especially with professors that you feel you jive particularly well with.

The mistake that most students make is forgetting that office hours even exist until the last few weeks of the semester, or until the week before an exam. Chances are, everyone will want to see the professor during those times, which won't leave a lot of opportunity for you to work your magic and make a new professor-friend. Again, the earlier in the semester that you start reaching out (and the more you keep it up, even in semesters where you are not taking one of their classes), the more likely they will be to actually remember who you are when it comes time to write that letter. They will be more eager to put time and effort into this process for you, instead of just sending around the stock "She is a great student, attentive, and a joy to have in class" that probably has been said for about 100 of your peers and classmates.

Highlighting Your Diverse Interests and Skills

When making choices about certain recommenders, the thought process is similar to the one that should be driving your approach to the application as a whole: you are seeking to convey the diverse interests, skills, values, and interesting tidbits that make you who you are. If you are fortunate enough to have multiple professors to choose from who can write in detail about you, then you should choose carefully.

Here are a few things to keep in mind.

DO YOUR RESEARCH

When you start thinking about who should write your letters, make sure to ground your search in the requirements outlined on the websites of your goal schools. Most schools will require anywhere between four and six letters of recommendation. The things that may differ include whether they require one or some to be from a specific department, such as from a science course, from a professor in the department that awarded your major, or from your school's pre-med "committee." It is important to know what these requirements are so that you can strategically plan the process of finding the ideal people.

GO FOR VARIETY

As you are a diverse person with a multitude of skills and interests, you want a gamut of recommendation letters that will reflect that variety. That means you should try to pick professors from classes in different fields. For example, the professor from your fiction writing class may be able to speak to your creativity and the way you speak up in your seminars with ease and confidence. On the other hand, the professor who taught you biochemistry may be able to comment on the quality of the questions that you ask in class, how you are consistently prepared for the lesson, and that you are curious about more in-depth material. An easy rule of thumb is to have at least one recommender who teaches a STEM course and at least one who teaches a course in the social sciences. If you can nail down those two, you have a lot more flexibility in determining who else to ask.

BRANCH OUT

Don't limit yourself only to academic letters of recommendation. Actually, some schools will *require* that you submit from people who can speak to what contributions you can make outside of an academic context. Again, you would benefit from checking in with your goal schools to see if this is a requirement and, if it is, *obviously* invest in building some nonacademic relationships. Even if it is not a requirement, however, a letter from your supervisor in a lab, at work, or from the clinic that you volunteer at could still add another dimension to your application.

WHAT

After you've established who you will ask for letters, you want to think about managing what will actually go into your letter of recommendation. Even though you won't be the one writing it, you have a lot of power to wield here. Professors who agree to write letters for you, even if they know you and can write confidently about your personality, probably don't know a whole lot about you outside the context of their class or lab. This is especially true in larger schools, where professors may have up to 500 students on their roster each semester.

For that reason, anyone who agrees to write a recommendation letter for you will often ask you to write a description about yourself and your academic trajectory up to this point. They will also request that you send them an updated résumé. This is a perfect opportunity for you to highlight what is important to you, what you enjoy learning about, and why this particular class/lab experience has been meaningful on your path to medicine.

Even if they don't request that supplementary material from you, you are better off sending it, just in case. Every professor is a person with a life and a long list of commitments, of which your recommendation letter is only one. Chances are, your professor has already written hundreds of letters throughout his/her career and therefore has *tons* of stock material to pull from if they get stuck or need some fillers. Filling in those gaps for them, in your own words about experiences, values, and traits that are specific to you as an applicant, will decrease the chances that they will dip into their "stock" when writing your letter. This will help you to stand out as an applicant. Ideally, you will be able to tailor your supplementary material and résumé for each recommender, so each letter will highlight different strengths and traits to help paint a complete picture of you as an applicant and medical school hopeful.

For example, if you received a C in one of your classes, but feel you showed the professor what a diligent, hard worker you can be because you were always in office hours demonstrating how much you care, that professor may talk about your grit and perseverance in the face of challenging material. Your request for that letter might look something like this. I am writing it in email form, but never underestimate the power of an in-person meeting. Use email as a backup in case you are off-campus or you are under a tight deadline.

Dear Professor WhoGaveMeaC,

I wanted to thank you so much for an incredible semester! I really enjoyed your class and found that your teaching style and willingness to answer all of my questions helped me to understand the material much better than I would have on my own. While my final grade in this course was not as high as I would have hoped, I was wondering if you would be willing to write a recommendation letter for me for medical school. I believe that despite this low outcome, I was able to show my commitment to understanding the material and am proud of the effort I put forth in your class.

I would welcome the opportunity to chat more about this request in person if you have any availability next week.

Best,
Elisabeth

The reason I am spending so much time on this scenario is that people tend to gravitate toward professors of the classes in which they are most successful. While it is awesome that you have those courses, it is also really important that your professor can write something other than, "I taught Elisabeth in Genetics, and can confirm that she got an A. She is clearly a very bright student and I enjoyed working with her."

Now don't get me wrong. That is all perfectly nice, but again, it doesn't tell an adcom anything about you that they don't already know from the transcript you have submitted. A letter like that is a wasted opportunity to let the adcom know something more meaningful about you besides that you were successful in a science course (a trait which almost every competitive applicant with a shot of getting into medical school also shares). You want your letters to contain information that will help you stand out from the crowd of your peers, so never be shy in making that information *readily* available and accessible for your recommender.

Similarly, you want to choose someone who can speak to you as a person, a student, and a future doctor. That also means someone who is willing and able to commit the time that it takes to write a really strong letter of recommendation for you. A mistake that a lot of people make is trying to get the "flashiest" recommenders (e.g., the Nobel Prize winner sitting in your university's Physics department who doesn't teach any classes but who is technically listed as the professor of your Physics 101 course). While name dropping is cool, you are much better off having that person's doctoral student write you a recommendation letter than you are getting what will undoubtedly be a stock letter from the man himself.

WHEN

So we have talked about who to ask and what kind of information to include about yourself to help guide your recommender toward a tailored and personalized representation of who you are. What we have not touched on yet is when to ask recommenders for those letters.

Ideally, you want to get on their radar by requesting a recommendation letter during a time when you are still fresh in their memory. Professors will have hundreds of students in any given year, and once you no longer see them day-to-day, the harder it will be for them to write about your abilities and skills in a way that is detailed, honest, and persuasive.

Let's look at why you will want to ask for recommendation letters from professors in your junior and senior year of college, or during a post-bac program.

UPPER-LEVEL CLASSES

Professors (for the most part) don't like teaching Intro classes, but do like teaching upper-levels. They tend to design and teach upper-levels in classes that align with their own research and that include topics in which they are interested. This makes them more likely to *want* to converse with you about the topics you are learning. They usually dislike introductory level courses so much (the information is rudimentary, the students are just starting to get into their groove and don't actually even know if they are interested in the material) that most of them tend to assign the actual teaching of the course to advanced graduate and doctorate students. Also, there is a lot of material that simply *must* be covered in an introductory course in order for students to have the knowledge to move on to more advanced courses in the department. This does not give professors a lot of flexibility to focus on their topics of interest or perceived importance. Conversely, professors often get to design upper-level courses around their areas of interest and expertise, and get to teach them to a small pool of students. These students are (likely) genuinely interested in the complex material covered by the course, and professors are definitely keen to chat with you about it if you convey that interest.

Myth: You should start asking professors for recommendation letters as soon as you step foot on your college campus.

Moral: Upper-level courses often available to third- and fourth-year students are ideal settings for building connections with potential recommenders.

APPLICATION TIMING

Your junior and senior years are much closer to the time of your application than your freshman and sophomore years. That means the letters you request later on in the application process are more likely to reflect the type of student that you will be when you matriculate to medical school, which is exactly what admissions committees are interested in learning about you as you apply.

A BETTER STUDENT

You are more likely to be a better student by your third year of college, and may therefore be more successful in classes—something that never hurts when you are asking for a letter!

Again, there is no law to say that you should only get letters of recommendations from professors in whose classes you excelled. However, most students are on an "upward trajectory" in terms of academic performance between their first and last years of college. For example, in my freshman year, I took an elective course taught by the professor who ultimately became my advisor. I ended up getting a B+ in the class—respectable, but not great for my medical school aspirations. In my junior year, I took a class by the same professor and received an A+. Quite a jump numerically. However, the most important piece of that difference was the way in which my professor perceived me as a student. He had never been shy in letting me know that he thought I was flighty upon first meeting me, and was largely unsure how long my desire to go to medical school would last. For this reason, he did not accept me into his lab as a first-year student. However, by the time I took my second class with him, my work ethic and commitment to both mastering and advancing in the subject matter was clear to him (or so he says). The progress impressed him and he wrote about it in his recommendation letter for me. At that point, he was able to honestly report that he was convinced of my commitment to attending and excelling in medical school.

For academic letters of recommendation, building relationships with your professors is important, but don't stress about it until later in your college career. For nonacademic letters, the sooner you can start diving into research projects, work, or volunteering that really speaks to your interests, the more relationships you will build with your supervisors that may lead to letters of recommendation.

How

The last piece of this recommendation letter puzzle is the actual process of requesting the letter. This request will (hopefully) stimulate an important transaction, in which a professor who knows and respects you will donate his or her time and energy to support your candidacy to medical school.

The important thing to remember here is that professors are not obligated to write a letter of support for you. They are encouraged to write letters in general as part of their professional responsibilities, but the commitment to write a letter for *you* is a personal favor to *you*. You want to be respectful of that fact as you ask them for this favor.

IN-PERSON MEETINGS

Ask to schedule an in-person meeting with them to discuss your request. Ideally, you want to be alone with this person so that you can have their undivided attention about this serious matter. Email them to set up a time to chat, and be clear that you want to chat about a *request for* a recommendation letter. Then, propose a few times to meet, either during or directly before/after their office hours. You want to make this as convenient as possible for them. Meeting in person will also help them put a face to a name, which is something that most professors will undoubtedly appreciate.

Give them a lot of information about who you are, what you've done, and what role the recommendation letter will serve in your application. Ideally, upon leaving that in-person discussion, you will have outlined a plan with your professor that will include three important dates:

1. when they can expect an email from you with information about yourself and your accomplishments,

2. when you would like them to have the recommendation letter submitted (my recommendation is about a month before it is officially "due"), and

3. finally, the absolute *last* date they can submit before their letter is delaying your application.

Let's talk about each of these.

ALL ABOUT YOU

As I've mentioned before, most professors will ask you to provide them with a "quick sheet" of information about you and what qualities or skills it is most helpful for them to write about. Now don't get me wrong, I am not proposing that you send an email that says "Please write about my excellent leadership abilities," because that would be both rude and quite unethical. However, if you send an email that includes a list of activities, including "President of Club X," that might give your professor a segue to talk about the leadership abilities you exhibited in his class. Similarly, you don't want to say "Please remind adcoms that I got an A in this class," but you could say something along the lines of "My performance in STEM classes has improved greatly over the last few years, and I would be grateful if you could highlight that by mentioning the success I have enjoyed in your class."

DEADLINES

Giving professors a "soft" deadline can be very beneficial for you as an applicant equest and can alleviate a lot of the stress that comes with waiting for a recommendation letter pack to reach your schools after you have already submitted. Some professors may even be grateful for the deadline, particularly if you ask during the summer months when professors plan to submit their own research for publication. However, don't ask them to submit in March when they know applications don't open until June. That unnecessary pressure can be frustrating, so respectfully suggest they try to submit a few weeks before applications open. Additionally, if you have a fall-semester class with a professor, request them to complete their letter as early as possible. This allows them to knock one letter out of the way before the barrage of requests comes in, and gives them the flexibility to simply upload an already written document when the time comes. Plus, they will have your performance in recent memory. You also want to be as communicative as possible with them—something as simple as "*Would it be helpful if I sent a reminder to you about this the week before my deadline?*" This can help you both manage your expectations and relieve pressure on a professional who likely has several things on his or her plate already.

MISSING DEADLINES

Budget for one professor missing the deadline or forgetting to write the letter for you. An incredibly important detail to remember about this entire process is that schools will NOT look at partially completed applications. This means that even though you will have taken all the fabulous advice in this book and submitted your application on the day that applications open in June, it won't matter if your professors are not similarly diligent in holding up their end of the bargain. This may happen for a variety of reasons. Maybe they overcommitted for letters and you have not been as diligent about reminding them as some of your peers, maybe they were too busy with their own work or maybe they simply forgot that they agreed to do it. This means that if your school has a system for "storing" letters that professors write (i.e., a committee letter process that combines all the letters you have received into a letter pack that will get sent to all of your schools), it may behoove you to ask for one more letter than you actually need. Similarly, if your schools ask for four to six recommendation letters, prepare yourself to have more than the minimum number of letters. I cannot think of anything worse than your application being delayed because someone else failed to deliver on their word; however, pity about an unfortunate situation will not help you get into medical school, so it is best to be prepared from the start.

Remember that it is on you to make this process as easy as possible for professors who are often already overcommitted due to the nature of their work. Take the time to get to know them so they are not trying to remember who you are, provide them with all the information they request (and more) in a timely manner, and send appropriately spaced reminder emails to help them if needed. Ultimately, the responsibility to meet the requirement for letters of recommendation is yours, and you should not depend on anyone else for ensuring it gets done.

DESIGNING YOUR SCHOOL LIST | 9

While each medical school will teach you roughly the same content, the experiences that you will have at each will be incredibly different. You will want to apply to somewhere between 15 and 20 medical schools (the national average is a whopping 16 applications per person). When determining what your list is going to look like, your MCAT score and GPA will be important players. After all, you want to apply to at least a couple of schools where your candidacy will be very competitive and where you are likely to be admitted. However, there is great variation in culture, experience, and curriculum, even among schools who admit similar candidates.

Because so many schools have similar GPA and MCAT ranges for incoming students, it is possible that your scores will make you competitive for admission at far more than 16 schools. You will need a strategy for whittling that down to a manageable number.

Now you may be wondering why you should limit yourself to less than 20 medical schools. I mean, if this is a highly competitive process and there is a chance that you won't be admitted to a school, even if your application is better than average, doesn't it make statistical sense to maximize your chances by increasing your number of submitted applications? Logically, yes. You would be absolutely correct to want to apply to all 141 MD programs and 34 DO programs in the country. However, there are three key limitations that make this strategy impractical.

1. Each primary application you submit will cost you an $170 for the verification process and $39 per school to which it is sent.

2. Each school will require you to write between one and seven additional essays in order to complete their secondary application. You will have to do that. There will also be some, albeit in some cases artificial, time constraints on how long you will get to do that. Plus, schools will have secondary application fees as high as $150 required for your application to progress.

3. The last page of your AMCAS application (the one that gets sent to all of your schools) will be a list of all the schools to which you have applied. Adcoms will be wary of students who have applied to too many schools, as it is an indication that that student has not researched what medical schools are best-fit schools and is perhaps not ready to begin the application process at all. In a survey conducted for this book, admissions officers from more than 50 medical schools across the country were asked to quantify how many schools is *too* many for an applicant to have applied to. Unsurprisingly, the results clustered between 18 and 22. No one answered a number under 14, and six respondents said that 25+ is too many schools.

The bottom line is that you want to be selective to which schools you give your time and money. Aside from the financial cost of applying to medical school, I can't quite explain the unsettling feeling you get in the pit of your stomach as you sit down on August 24 to begin writing a 3,000-word essay about your childhood with an August 26 deadline for a school that you aren't even really sure you would want to go to even if they did accept you. Oh, and did I mention that by that time, you will have been writing secondaries every single day since the beginning of July?

This is an emotionally draining process—the least you can do for yourself is make sure that all the schools you are doing this for are schools that would actually be worth your effort.

If you were the average applicant in the United States in the 2018 application cycle, you would have applied to 16 schools. We'll use that as our goal as we work through how to come up with your list.

First School

The first school on your list should be your state school (or the school that your state has reciprocity with if your state of residence is Alaska, Delaware, Montana, or Wyoming). While the exact percentages vary state by state, admissions rates are highest across the board for in-state residents at state universities. Since the chances of the average applicant being accepted to his/her state school are statistically best this is a good one to add to your list.

Reciprocity or Linkage Program

If your undergraduate school has a reciprocity or a linkage program with a medical school, or if it is well known that a medical school accepts a high percentage of students from its undergraduate institution (as is true for Johns Hopkins University and the Johns Hopkins School of Medicine), that would be another great one to add to your list. Again, we are trying to play the odds in a very competitive game.

Remaining Schools

For your 14 remaining schools, you will want to take a look at the MSAR, or the Medical School Admissions Requirements. You will need to purchase access to this tool from the AAMC, but the one-year access you get for $28 will tell you everything you need to know about accepted student GPA and MCAT data; relevant medical, volunteer and/or research experiences of accepted students; tuition and financial aid information; and much more for all U.S. and Canadian medical schools. Using your actual or projected MCAT scores and GPA, you can see which schools you should apply to in order to increase your chances for admission. Use the following steps to help determine the rest of your school list.

1. Pick six schools for which at least one of your numbers is above the average of accepted students (you are in the 75th percentile of accepted students).

2. Pick five schools for which your numbers are at or slightly below the average of accepted students (you are between the 25th and 50th percentile of accepted students).

3. Pick three schools for which your numbers are below the average of accepted students (you are below the 25th percentile of accepted students)—these schools are what you probably called "reach" schools in your college application process.

You can modulate those numbers slightly, depending on how strong the remainder of your application is. For example, if you have been a lead author on a paper published in a large peer-reviewed journal, you will likely be safe adding a few more schools in your "reach" category.

Conversely, if your numbers are not above the 50th percentile for any MD schools, you may want to consider one of the following options to increase your chances of admission:

1. Pursue some post-graduate coursework to get your GPA up

2. Retake the MCAT in hopes of improving your score

3. Consider applying to newer medical schools (<5 years old) that likely have fewer applicants than a school that is more established

If it is still early on in your college career and you have ample opportunity to change what your numbers will look like by the time you apply, use the MSAR as a goal-setting tool. The world is your oyster! Think about where you want to go and what you need to do in school to make that happen.

If you keep all we've mentioned so far in mind, you will manage to whittle your list down *a little bit,* based on your qualifications alone. However, the point is not only that you get accepted to medical school, but also that you are accepted to a school that you would be happy attending, and whose curriculum is designed in a way that is conducive to your success. After all, medical school is only a pit stop on your way to the ultimate goal of becoming a practicing doctor, There is no use in attending a school where you won't be able to succeed.

Here are some other things to consider as you're researching medical schools.

Academic Day-to-Day

How do they grade? Pass/fail or letter grades? Are lectures required attendance? When are labs and tests scheduled? Are exams scheduled on Fridays or Mondays, and do you prefer to have the weekend off or the weekend to study? What proportion of your learning will be lecture style vs. small group work? How stressed are the students at this school? Are they competitive or friendly amongst themselves?

These things might sound like small details, but the answers to these questions will determine what your next four years will look like and are definitely worth considering as you decide where to apply.

Broader Values and Performance

Is the school a stronger research university or a stronger primary care university? Are dual degrees available? How many electives will you have to complete in order to graduate? Do they have nonacademic requirements, like research or community service? Do they have programs and opportunities for minority students? How many weeks do they set aside for USMLE prep in Year 2? How do students from this school perform on the USMLE? Where are they matching for residency? How much flexibility do students have in designing their schedule? How comfortable is the administration with granting time off for health/other pursuits?

Geography

Is the school in an urban, suburban, or rural environment? How affordable is it to live near the school? Will you need a car while you're there to get to rotations? What hospitals do they work with, and subsequently, what kind of exposure are students getting in third and fourth year? What type of patient population does the University Hospital predominantly serve? How close is the school to your family, friends, and support network?

Chances are you won't be able to find a school that checks all of your boxes, but it is worth identifying which of these are most important to you and aiming for schools that fit with your preferences across these categories.

When I applied to medical school, I made the mistake of basing my school list almost solely on rankings and on how well-known the schools were. As I progressed in the process and had received some acceptances, I was able to be more selective in the schools that I travelled to for the interview. In doing so, I realized how poorly I had conducted my school search the first time around, and how little I had considered the issues that "fit" me.

For example, geography is probably the most important lever on that list for me. I knew that I would not be able to spend four years living happily in a rural area. I need to be in a city, where I have outlets for hobbies and a social life, and where I can easily travel when given the opportunity. However, I still spent (read: might as well have *burned*) $567 sending primary and secondary applications to schools in rural areas.

I didn't realize this until I received two different interview invitations in different parts of the country for the same week. The way the dates had worked out, I was not able to go to both, and was thus forced to *really* consider which of those schools I would be least happy attending. I ultimately decided to decline the invitation to a school whose values, curriculum, and dual-degree options were absolutely perfect for me, but that was located in an extremely rural area in the northeast. After scouring my network for a current student to contact, I asked how he spends his time out of class, and he answered, "Well, you won't have much honestly, but when you do have some free time, a lot of people hike, ski, and do other outdoorsy things."

Well, that was that. I am not exactly the outdoorsy type and you would definitely *not* call me athletic. As much as I tried, I simply couldn't picture spending four years of my life in a place where all my leisure time would be filled with nature.

Not applying to this school and others sharing similar surrounding environments would have:

- saved me a lot of time and money on the front end (I mean let's face it, it's not like I was Miss Nature in June and suddenly changed when I got the interview invitation); and

- given me the opportunity to explore and find schools in urban areas that could have potentially worked for me.

To save yourself from making these same costly mistakes, run each of the schools you are thinking of applying to through the following filters:

- Can I get in?

- Can I thrive there academically?

- Is this an institution that will prioritize/care about my mental and emotional well-being?

- Is this school located somewhere where I would want to spend the next four years?

- And finally, can I afford it? We will discuss this filter in greater detail in the next chapter.

PAYING FOR THE APPLICATION AND MEDICAL SCHOOL | 10

THE APPLICATION

Applying to medical school is expensive, with the average applicant committing over $2,800 from the time they submit their primary to the time they matriculate. I won't lie to you—it will be challenging without parental support, but there are some ways to at least minimize costs as much as possible.

If you are reading this as a freshman or sophomore in college, you may be in a position to start proactively saving for the application process, which may be harder to finance than medical school tuition. While there will be numerous scholarship and loan opportunities available to you when you have your acceptance in hand, the application process itself is expensive, and financial supports are available to a smaller range of students. While I wish I were in a position to change that reality, I am settling for second best here: giving you a clear picture of all the costs you will face so that money will not keep you from completing all of these moving pieces on time.

MSAR ACCESS

As we move through the process chronologically, the first medical school-specific resource you will want to purchase is access to the MSAR, the Medical School Admissions Requirements. This online database gives you detailed information about every U.S. and Canadian MD-granting and LCME-accredited medical school, as well as some baccalaureate-MD programs. This resource will be useful in helping you build your school list based on which schools fit what you are looking for, as well as which are likely to accept you. It also has some other fancy functionalities, such as creating comparisons between schools and syncing to your calendar to track important deadlines for primary and secondary applications (although for most schools, there are much more important unspoken deadlines that you should aim toward). One-year access to the MSAR database will set you back $28.

MCAT

As you begin to prepare for the MCAT, you will likely incur some costs for books, materials, prep courses, and/or tutors. These can vary in costs from $25 to thousands of dollars, depending on how much external support you need.

PREPARING FOR THE TEST

Some resources that you might want to consider purchasing include:

- AAMC-published full-length practice exams, which give you a sense of how you might score on the real thing: $268 for the Official MCAT Prep Bundle

- A book set from your favorite test-prep company, which will give you guidance on what material to focus on as you prepare for the exam: $250 average for six books

- Tutoring or class packages from your favorite test-prep company: packages range from $150–$2,500 on average

- To save yourself some of these costs, Khan Academy has partnered with the AAMC to create MCAT-specific content videos and ~150 practice passages

REGISTERING FOR THE TEST

Without factoring in late registration or cancellation fees, it costs between $305 and $370 to sit for the MCAT, depending on when you register for the test. Ideally, you will be able to register at a testing site near your home, but if not, you may have to factor in some travel costs. Fortunately, the available testing sites are fairly well distributed across the country. But if you are in a rural area and know there aren't a lot of testing sites near you, you will want to prioritize registering for the test as soon as it becomes available. In January and August, which are the most popular testing months, this fact will be even more important. While this travel issue will probably not be a huge deal for you, it could be. When the new version of the MCAT was released in March 2015, the last two test dates for the old version of the test were in January 2015. Wary about having to study for a fourth section, having to sit for a longer test, and being in the first batch of new scores, everyone that could scrambled to take those January tests. At one point, people were actually purchasing plane tickets to Hawaii, Alaska, and Montana, the last sites with any space, just to take their MCAT!

Additionally, MCAT test takers outside the United States, Canada, Guam, the U.S. Virgin Islands, and Puerto Rico will also pay an additional international registration fee of $105.

CANCELING OR RESCHEDULING

Registering more than two weeks before your test can save you $50 on registration fees alone. What's more, early registration also gives you cheaper rescheduling fees for test date or location, and a greater refund in case of cancellation. Now don't get too excited—the maximum cancellation refund is $150, and the cheapest rescheduling fee is $75, no matter how early you register. Definitely not great bang-for-your-buck, but better than nothing, I guess. You want to make sure to get in that sweet spot of early enough to avoid any late fees, but within striking distance, so you can arrange a reasonable study schedule based on what your life will actually look like as you prepare for this exam. To avoid any cancellation or rescheduling fees, you want to be as intentional and organized as possible when you decide to register. You should also be honest with yourself and know how long you will need to prepare. Having to incur a rescheduling or cancellation fee on top of an already expensive exam is incredibly frustrating. However, it will still be cheaper to pursue either of these options if you aren't prepared than it will be to have to re-take the exam. Not to mention, it will help you avoid having a poor score on your application.

APPLICATION FEES

There are several fees associated with the application itself.

AMCAS FEES

The primary application is the first thing sent via AMCAS to all of your schools. The initial fee of $170 will cover the cost of AMCAS processing and verifying your application. This will also cover the cost of AMCAS forwarding that completed application to *one* school. There will then be a $39 cost for sending that application to each additional school.

SECONDARY FEES

Almost every school you apply to will be sending you a secondary application to fill out, with questions specific to their school, programs, and values. The exception to this is the small proportion of schools who will pre-screen applicants and only send secondary applications to the students that fit their academic criteria. After you spend hours crafting these essays, you will also get to pay the school somewhere between $75 and $150 to submit the secondary application to them. Yes, that will happen for each and every school you want to submit a secondary to, and no, secondaries are unfortunately not optional if you wish your application to progress any further.

TIP

Take a look at your "reach" schools and find out if they pre-screen applicants. If you are significantly below their 50th percentile of accepted students, you may not reach their threshold for a secondary application, and thus won't even want to spend the money on the primary application. If you are unsure, it is worth a quick phone call to that school's admissions office to see if you can get an honest answer about your chances there.

TIP

The unwritten rule for secondary applications is that you want to submit them within two weeks after they are sent to you. If you can, try to have at least some of those funds set aside before secondary season even begins. Once it starts, not only will you have three essays to submit to each school, but you also will likely receive all of your secondary application invitations around the same time (this is potentially more like three essays × 16 schools!) You don't want to have to worry about coming up with the cash to send in your secondaries on top of that, if you can avoid it.

MISCELLANEOUS

In addition to these rather hefty costs, there are some smaller ones that may also add up, including the fees to get your transcripts from your school to AMCAS, or a one-time fee to someone to read over your application if you need some additional feedback.

INTERVIEW

After a few (very) expensive summer months, you will have anywhere from a few weeks to a few months of radio silence from all of your schools. On their end, this is a time of reading applications and deliberating about who they will invite to interview. If finances are of particular concern to you, this would be a good time to prepare saving for potential interviews that may come up. The AAMC estimates that the typical applicant will spend about $4,500 during one interview season on travel, lodging, and interview attire. Plus, if you work, you will have to factor in the potential lost income during the days you will be travelling.

> **TIP**
>
> If you receive interview invitations from schools that are in the same geographical area, reach out to those schools to see if they will work with you so you only have to make one trip. This is also a good excuse to get in touch if you have not heard back from them yet. Something like, "I currently live in Texas but will make the trip to New England in the second week of November for an interview. I have not received an invitation to interview yet from you, but if there is any way to know whether or not I might, and whether planning it for that same week might be possible, I would be greatly appreciative," is a polite way to start a conversation surrounding your prospects. It also has the potential to save you a lot on travel costs. Granted, the answer might be a polite-but-firm "no," but it never hurts to ask.

Post-Acceptance

Besides the obvious expense of tuition that will come up once you receive that coveted acceptance letter, there are also some other pesky expenses that could incur even after you've come home from the interview, particularly if you are holding more than one acceptance.

- **Acceptance deposits:** In order to hold a place at a medical school until May, you may be required to give an acceptance deposit. You may need this time if you are waiting to hear back from other schools or are trying to decide where to attend. The deposits can vary from school to school, but probably won't be cheap. For example, the medical school deposit at Georgetown University is $500.

- **Accepted student days:** Again, if you are in the fabulous position of having been accepted to more than one medical school, you may want to attend an Accepted Student or Second Look Day to get a better idea of the school. This means there will likely be some travel costs that can add up fairly quickly.

The most frustrating thing about this list of costs is that, barring the post-interview list, there are unfortunate consequences associated with not having the money to complete each part of the application. Ian from California spoke to me about making the difficult decision to delay his application by a year because he felt the application delays, brought about by the financial strain of the process, would have made his application less competitive.

> *"I had no parental support going through college and had worked all four years of undergrad to pay for housing, books, and transportation. I had also taken out student loans to pay for the part of my tuition that was not covered by federal grants or financial aid. I thought I was*

*doing pretty well, honestly, but didn't
expect the cost of the application to be so
high. Anyway, to make a long story short,
I ended up getting sick for two weeks in
July and not being able to work, leaving
me short about $1,500. I obviously
had to pay for rent and food first, and
had already maxed out my credit card
paying for the primary application the
previous month. I had about $92 in my
bank account and was offered another
$100 from my parents for help. That
would have been enough for maybe two
secondary applications, if I picked my
schools wisely. I just didn't think that was
enough, so I ended up having to go in and
withdraw from each school. I'm currently
in the process of saving up money so that
I can apply this cycle—I'm aiming for
about $2,000, and then I'll think about
the interview costs when that time comes."*

If you find yourself in a position similar to Ian's, you may
qualify for the AAMC's Fee Assistance Program. The FAP
is dependent upon financial needs and offers a reduced

MCAT registration fee, complimentary MSAR access, a waiver for AMCAS fees for one application submission with up to 20 school designations, and, if applicable, up to an $800 benefit toward an updated psychoeducational or medical re-evaluation if it is necessary to support your MCAT accommodations application.

FINANCING MEDICAL SCHOOL

Obviously medical school is expensive. So was undergrad. This section will talk a little bit about to how to pay for these upcoming expenses. The largest expense associated with medical school is, of course, the tuition. However, there are also other costs, such as housing, transportation (especially if you need it to get to/from school or rotations in your third and fourth years), and "small" miscellaneous things, such as your laptop, the cost of sitting for Step 1, and health insurance.

If you have parental financial support through this process and will not have to take out a full loan, you should put this book down right now and thank your parents. Otherwise, you will likely be doing some combination of:

- financing your cost of attendance on your own through your own savings;
- working through medical school to cover cost of living and small miscellaneous expenses; and
- taking out student loans or getting scholarships.

If you are planning to (even partially) finance your cost of attendance, you may consider taking a gap year in order to save up some cash through a full-time job. If you are planning to work while in medical school, you should tread carefully. Any first-year student you speak to will tell you that the first semester is overwhelming, due to the breadth of material you are charged with learning and the depth of knowledge required to be successful. Keep this in mind as you plan a schedule that includes work, especially if you have no financial fallback in case your nonacademic load begins infringing on your academic performance.

You can also limit any high-cost surprises by proactively looking into the *total cost of attendance* annually (not just tuition) for schools that interest you, and to prioritize your application to low-cost universities. *U.S. News and Report* publishes a list of the least expensive medical schools every year.

Financial Aid and Scholarships

If you are planning on taking out student loans, consider the implications of lifetime limits on subsidized loans, and the future financial implications of taking out unsubsidized or private loans. According to the Free Application for Federal Student Aid (FAFSA), the subsidized and unsubsidized aggregate loan limit (including loans incurred in undergraduate programs) is $138,500 for graduate or professional students, and no more than $65,500 of this amount may be in subsidized loans. The graduate aggregate limit includes all federal loans received for undergraduate study.

While you will likely be making a comfortable salary as a doctor, student loan debt of this magnitude is something that will be with you potentially for years after graduation. Make sure you speak with your parents, counselors, mentors, and potentially a financial advisor before deciding to take this on. Here are some other options you could consider as well:

- Thousands of students each year apply for the Health Professions Scholarship Program (HPSP). Sponsored by the U.S. Army, Navy, and Air Force, this scholarship covers 100% of tuition and supplies and provides a monthly stipend for living expenses. In exchange, you will be required to serve on active duty one year for each year of support you receive.

- The National Health Service Corps Scholarship will similarly provide tuition, fees, and any other educational costs in addition to a small stipend for living expenses. Recipients will commit to completing a residency in either family medicine, internal medicine, pediatrics, OB/GYN, or psychiatry and to practicing medicine in a designated high-need urban, rural, or frontier site. The service commitment is one year for each year of support you receive and has a two-year minimum commitment.

- Residents of Alaska, Arizona the Commonwealth of the North Mariana Islands, Colorado, Hawaii,

Montana, Nevada, New Mexico, North Dakota, Utah, and Wyoming are also eligible to apply to the Professional Student Exchange Program (PSEP). Participating geographies offer support to students attending professional programs that are not available at public institutions in their home state.

For all of these options, make sure to look into important deadlines for application, and consider all commitments and requirements.

COMPLETING YOUR SECONDARY APPLICATIONS | 11

The summer you decide you are ready to apply to medical school will look something like the following.

1. June: Submission of primary application, wave of relief, feeling of overwhelming accomplishment.

2. Four to six weeks of radio silence while AMCAS processes and verifies your application.

3. A single secondary application invitation comes in. This is it. The time has come, sh*t is getting real, you are really doing this. Revel in it. *Dream School likes me enough to send me a secondary application.*

Swoon

24–28 HOURS LATER

All the other secondary requests start pouring in. You go to take a shower and your email is blowing up. You would feel excited and popular if you weren't so overwhelmed about how you're going to write all these essays and fill out all these forms and keep all these passwords straight. Some applications have explicit deadlines. Some don't, but you know better than to believe that. You have 43 essays and short answer responses to write over the next 14 days.

You make yourself some coffee and sit down to start. All memories of your childhood seem to be gone. You get asked to enter the details of all your completed coursework (Didn't I do this already? Didn't AMCAS verify it? What are they trying to do, catch a mistake?).

1. Proceed to question whether medical school is really worth it.

2. Quick break to research other career paths. Briefly freak out about how little else you are qualified to do.

3. Cry.

4. Get back to writing.

Repeat for the next two to four weeks

The primary application, which included your personal statement, transcript, letters of recommendation, and activities list, is what you sent to AMCAS for processing, verification, and distribution to the schools of your choice. All of that information goes to each and every school you apply to, and thus only has to be submitted once.

The secondary applications, on the other hand, are the source of all the madness described above because they are medical-school-specific applications. That means that each medical school has its own questions and information it wants to know about you. It will send you its own set of questions for you to answer, that you will then send directly to the school itself through your unique portal. The questions will vary in length and content, but will largely have you discussing yourself, your family, your journey to medicine, your passion for medicine, your thoughts about your future career as a physician, and why you are so excited about embarking on your personal journey with this particular school as your starting point.

And the best part about it all is that all of the questions are just *slightly* different enough that you won't be able to just copy and paste a full response from one text box to another.

If it seems overwhelming now, just wait until they're all coming at you at the same time.

Here are some strategies and tips for avoiding the crazy while keeping your competitive edge:

SECONDARY STRATEGIES

There is an unspoken rule that you should turn your secondaries around two weeks after receiving them (at most). Schools know you are receiving between 10 and 20 requests for secondary applications within the same week. Most schools choose not to screen applications and thus send secondary requests to everyone with a verified primary, which means the numbers of requests are expected to be fairly high. Logic dictates that you will prioritize submitting secondaries for the schools that interest you most, so turning those around quickly can be another way to show your excitement for the school.

The average medical school secondary application has between one and nine essays for you to complete, with an average of four. Let's just think about that for a second. Even if you are the exception (which you won't be, but for the sake of argument, let's pretend) and *all* of your schools request only one response on their secondary applications and you apply to the 2018 average of 16 schools. You are still looking at writing *more than one essay response per day* in order to submit everything within the two-week window. And they have to be good. And you have to proofread them. And you have to make sure the information is consistent with what you put in your primary. Oh, and did I mention? *You* are the topic of interest for all of these essays!

Have you ever had to do that before? Write one essay a day for two straight weeks? It's not very fun. So, then what? Do you just have to resign yourself to this torture?

Secondary applications don't change much from year to year, and the prompts are available online for you to work through either during that period of radio silence, or even before you submit the primary. Start writing these early, as soon as you submit your primary application and have your school list. Chris from Maryland says, "The earlier you can start these steps, the more comfort you'll have when you reach that two-week sprint to turn around all the secondaries."

Angela from Tennessee recommends that you "Look online for prompts and then work through the most common ones first to maximize efficiency." Finally, you may find yourself having to make some tough choices about responding to all schools within the target window. Linda from Wyoming says, "You will be tempted to work through the secondaries in the order that they come in, but that isn't the best way. Spend an hour organizing your school list in order of preference, and work through secondaries in that order."

Do your research. Nothing will hurt you more than a generic response that shows you have no in-depth knowledge of the school or program to which you are applying.

ACING THE INTERVIEW | 12

YES! After months of anticipation, you *finally* get the invitation in your email and your heart skips a beat. You spend about five minutes figuring out what password you used for that school and finally log in to your account to pick the date for your much-awaited interview. Mark your calendar, buy your tickets and BOOM! Ready to go!

Congratulations, you have gotten past the toughest hurdle of the medical school application process, the one where the greatest proportion of applicants will get cut. You should be proud of yourself, as this is a tremendous feat. Schools have a limited number of interview invitations to give out and only extend those invitations to students in whom they are very interested.

So now that you've been placed on this short list, we want to make sure you can wow them in person. After all, that is what the interview is designed for: an opportunity for the admissions committee to get a sense of what drives you, what your personality is like, and what contribution you would make to their incoming class.

Preparing for your interview

Be Ready for the Questions You Will Definitely Be Asked

You should consider your interview for medical school admission no less formal or professional than an interview you would give to apply for a corporate job. In the survey we conducted in preparation for this book, the respondents said they spent an average of four hours and 20 minutes preparing for *each* of their medical school interviews. To determine what amount of time you should budget for preparation, you will need to do some introspection.

How confident are you thinking on your feet when asked a question? If you shudder at the very thought, you might want to increase the recommendation for these prep hours, just to be sure that you have at least some foundation for all the *types* of questions you will be asked. Of course, you will have to do some on-the-fly thinking because it is unlikely that you will be asked only questions that you are prepared to answer, but the more prepared you are ahead of time, the easier this will be.

If you rolled your eyes at that estimate, wondering how exactly anyone could spend over four hours preparing to answer a few short questions about *themselves,* I challenge you to consider the goal of the interview.

The interview is an opportunity to highlight that you are engaged, focused, mature, compassionate, committed to the study and practice of medicine, and an all-around nice person that your future professors, classmates, and patients would be happy interacting with on a daily basis. That's a pretty tall order for a half-hour slot of time! To do this most successfully, you want to make sure that you are giving a thoughtful, evidence-based, and succinct (no more than 45 seconds but no less than 20 seconds long) answer to any question that you are asked. Each answer should have a beginning, middle, and end, and ideally should call upon an example or experience you have had that informed your answer. You also need to make sure you address the *who, what, where, when, and how* of the short anecdote you will share, so that your interviewer can follow along. An effective way to prepare for this type of question is to come up with some stock anecdotes based on experiences you have had. Ideally, you could relate each of these to the "most valuable experiences" you listed on your primary application. These anecdotes should be reflective of the journey that you took before ultimately applying to medical school, and should top off with a brief explanation of why that experience impacted you and how it affected your medical school journey. Here are some examples of stock anecdotes that I had prepared:

- There was an unfortunate incident in my undergraduate research lab in which I forgot to heat my cell cultures and left them to die over the weekend. Thankfully, the impact was not detrimental to anyone else's work in the lab, and the cultures could be quickly remade. However, I learned from that experience that

I just couldn't be bothered to care about the fate of cells in a Petri dish. As horrible as that might sound to those of you committed to lab work, that revelation was tremendous for me. I was finally able to admit to myself that I was not passionate about pure lab-based work, and what intrigued me about medicine was the human interaction aspect. I really needed to visualize the impact of the science on human patients in order to commit my time and efforts to its progression. This then served as a jumping-off point for all volunteer work and social-science research I pursued for the rest of my college career.

- Then, there was the Saturday in the children's hospital where I met with a four-year-old girl who had become paralyzed after her family car was hit by a drunk driver. I had been chugging along in my pre-med career up to this point, fairly certain that I wanted to become a doctor. However, the guttural reaction I had when I saw this little girl in her wheelchair is what convinced me I *had* to be a doctor and had to do whatever possible in order to be useful to the next child that would come along.

- Finally, there was Melvin. The guy was exactly my age and had grown up less than five miles from me. However, Melvin grew up in a house with lead poisoning and had some learning difficulties that had caused him to drop out of high school at 16. Seeing him, a person that I could have met in other circumstances but didn't, or could have been friends with but wasn't, put a face on the social justice issues I had read about in the news. He compelled me to add a Social Policy minor to my degree.

After you figure out what anecdotes you want to speak about in the interview, write them out in little paragraphs. Then rehearse them until they are memorized and you can say them comfortably within a 45-second window. Keep rehearsing until you are so confident with this little monologue that it seems like you are coming up with the answers on the spot.

So how important is it that you prepare something like this, or that your answers are structured or fit into some defined amount of time? I mean, what are the chances that your interviews are going to be timed as you speak? (Zero, don't worry.) But let's take a look at how going into each question with this mindset can make you seem better prepared, more experienced, and an all-around stronger candidate than your peers.

No One-Word Answers

You walk into the interview room, sit down, and the interviewer tells you to relax and breathe. Some informal introductions are made and out of the way. Then they throw you that first question, the one that will set the tone for the rest of your interview. Let's say in this case it is "So, what type of doctor do you want to be?"

Easy-peasy right? Potentially a one-word answer. *Pediatrician. I want to be a pediatrician.* Fabulous. Question answered. Next?

No.

And here's why: a medical school interview is intended to be a conversation between you and your interviewer, where the interviewer gets to know you, and you get to learn about the school and potentially the interviewer's specific field of specialized medicine. Have you ever tried to have a conversation with someone who responds in curt, one-word answers? As an extreme extrovert and potentially one of the most talkative people you'd ever meet, I have. And while I have no problem continuing the conversation on my own, it is definitely not as fun as actually developing a bond with the person across the table from me.

An (almost) equally *bad answer* to that one-worded response would be something like: "I think I would like to be a pediatrician, but I'm not sure."

TIP

When preparing your interview answers, think about how the other person could respond to the answer you give.

What options have you just given your interviewer to continue your conversation? Not much other than a polite, "Oh, that's nice."

A medium answer might look something like this: "Well, I've volunteered a lot at my local children's hospital and really enjoyed that, so I think I would like to be a pediatrician."

You've added some additional information here, so at least there is something for your interviewer to latch onto to keep this conversation rolling. Additionally, you seemingly have put some thought into your answer because you are basing your response off of an experience you've had in the past. However, it does require *some* work and assumption-making on the part of your interviewer to come to that conclusion.

In contrast, a *good answer* might sound something like this: "While I'm sure this will change a lot as I proceed through medical school and gain more clinical exposure, if I had to pick a specialty tomorrow, I think I would choose to become a pediatrician. I have spent a total of about 300 hours volunteering at my local children's hospital over the last three years, and have really come to enjoy the different interactions I've had. Every child is so different, and it requires a certain combination of bribery, cajoling, and good humor to relate to them. Plus, there is a sense of joy and hope in pediatric wards that I think is lacking in wards with adult patients. So based on my experience thus far,

I think I can really see myself working in that field long-term."

So besides the obvious difference in length, what distinguishes these responses? I mean, they did all technically answer the question that the interviewer asked, right?

What Makes a Good Answer

Let's analyze what exactly makes this a good interview answer.

"While I'm sure this will change a lot as I proceed through medical school and gain more clinical exposure," shows that you are going into medical school with eyes wide open. You've acknowledged how much you still have to learn, but that you are interested in gaining this exposure.

"I have spent a total of about 300 hours volunteering at my local children's hospital over the last three years," calls attention to the experience that you do have. Yes, they already know this from your application, but highlighting volunteer experience that has shaped your perception of You-As-Doctor never hurts.

"Every child is so different, and it requires a certain combination of bribery, cajoling, and good humor to relate to them. Plus, there is a sense of joy and hope in pediatric wards that I think is lacking in wards with adult patients," shares something that you learned during all of those hours and places weight on this and future answers you will give.

"So based on my experience thus far, I think I can really see myself working in that field long-term," closes out your answer in a way that makes it clear you are finished speaking. It also helps you to avoid that thing when your voice gets quiet at the end of an answer or goes up in pitch as if you're asking a question. You know what I'm talking about? Both telltale signs that you are actually incredibly nervous being there.

A good tip for assessing the answers that you will draft and rehearse in preparation for your interviewers is to remember that the *content* of your answers is next to irrelevant. Your interviewer doesn't really care what specialty you think you'll want to pursue four years from now, because it isn't going to be relevant for another four years! What they are really looking for here is insight into how your brain works: what interests you, what catches your attention, and what experiences and feelings you felt were important enough to bring up.

Be Prepared for Controversial Questions

Doctors have to face patients with different political views than their own all the time and must treat them with respect and dignity regardless. To assess how well you may be able to do that in the future, as well as how receptive you are to new or challenging ideas, many adcoms have been known to ask opinion-based questions about controversial, medically related topics, like abortion or euthanasia.

Prepare for this to come up in your interview, with some introspection about what your opinion is on these and other similar topics. If you have a strong opinion in either direction, it is definitely appropriate to share if asked. However, make sure that you:

1. do so with respect to the opposing opinion and arguments;

2. recognize your responsibility as an aspiring physician to liaise with individuals sharing all kinds of political philosophies (and prejudices and opinions); and

3. are honest with your interviewer about the challenges that your position might raise for you in your practice and show that you have put some thought into how you might approach those challenges should they arise.

For example, let's say you are asked to defend your stance on abortion. A perfectly fine answer might explain that you are pro-life because a fertilized cell is, by definition, living, and that any termination of that pregnancy is something you consider to be unethical.

The matter of abortion is one that people can debate about and one that they have, in fact, debated about for decades in the United States. It's nice, respectable even, that you have an opinion on this very contentious issue one way or the other. However, a better approach to sharing that opinion in the setting of your medical school interview would be to discuss this issue through the lens of the physician-patient relationship. Remember, medicine is the ultimate service job. You will take an oath to serve the well-being of your patients under any circumstance. To highlight to your interviewer that you understand the weight of that responsibility, an answer like this might be more impactful:

> *"While I personally believe that abortion is unethical and is not the choice I would make for myself, my opinion on this matter is irrelevant. As a physician, I will owe it to my patient to respect any choice she makes within the legal guidelines. I do hope that I will be working in an environment wherein my views are respected and where I will be able to refer this patient to a colleague for the procedure itself, but I do recognize that I will have the responsibility to counsel and advise her as best I can regardless."*

While you are still giving an opinion here, you are also showing your interviewer that you have the critical thinking skills to acknowledge the merit in opinions different from your own, and the temperament to treat anyone who passes through your care with the dignity and respect he or she deserves.

Again, your interviewer does not really care *what* your opinion is either way, but rather whether and how it will affect your ability to practice medicine effectively. They want to know that you are thoughtful and mature enough to address one of the many potentially stressful situations that will you face in your career as a physician.

If you don't have an opinion on these or other possibly contentious issues that may come up in your interview, it would behoove you to spend some time learning about the common arguments fueling the debate. Raul, a biomedical engineering student who felt he wasn't informed enough to formulate an opinion on the eve of his medical school interviews, recommends listening to health and bioethics podcasts: "Google around a bit to see what interests you, and incorporate some informative podcasts into your daily commute so that you have some points to draw on in an interview."

Give Yourself an Attitude Check

If the point of the interview is to show the person sitting on the other side of the table that you are confident, competent, and ready for the emotional and mental roller coaster that is medical school, this is *not* the time to be nervous. Can we pause for a second to talk about the irony of this? That during what will likely feel like the most high-stakes conversations of your life, you will have to act like the ~kewlest kat~ there ever was. Annoying, I know—but completely doable! Here are some things you can chant to yourself as you do your power poses on the morning of:

- I would not be invited to this interview unless they already liked my application and wanted me to join their incoming class.

- I am interviewing this school and these people as much as they are interviewing me! Pfft. They should be the ones who are nervous.

- No one ever died from a med school interview.

- I know my stuff and can answer whatever questions come up! (You also want to make sure this last one is totally true, using the prepping suggestions outlined above.)

Finally, in addition to not being visibly nervous, you want to make sure you are not visibly arrogant. Your personality will dictate which side of confident you are more likely to lean to, but neither super nervous nor super arrogant are good places to be on interview day. If coming off as arrogant seems like a possibility for you, remind yourself that while yes, you are fantastic and obviously impressive (or you wouldn't have been invited to interview), so is everyone else that has been invited to interview. The goal is for the adcom to create a class of peers, students, and future doctors— arrogance is not a trait fit for any of those classifications.

Get As Much As You Can Out of Each Interview

Learn as much as you can about the school before you go to the interview, but know there there is a lot to learn during the interview itself as well. In addition to giving the school a sense of who you are and if you would be a good fit in their program, the interview day is also a great opportunity for you to get a sense of whether:

- you like the school,
- you like the surrounding area/where the school is located, and
- you can be successful there

If you are already going to commit the time, money, and energy required to interview at a medical school, you might as well make the most of that investment. Now, in a Maslow's-hierarchy-of-needs-type breakdown of the medical school admissions process, receiving an acceptance is obviously the base of the pyramid. Having to pick which school to attend based on how well the fit feels is a great problem to have. However, during your interview day, it is best to look past that little detail and prepare yourself to make a choice between two (or several) medical schools, should you be lucky enough to be in the position to do so.

Mike, an English major from Virginia, recommends you reach out to current students via the Admissions Office or your personal network. Would someone be able to host you if you are travelling? Would they be able to answer some questions for you over lunch or coffee? Chances are, you will find people to say "yes" to both, especially in schools where the students are happy and excited to be there. You also can address questions to current students that you can meet during your interview day (lunch with current students is fairly common) or with your interviewers. Here are some important things you might want to know, depending on what you prioritize in a medical school education and experience.

To get a sense of what your day-to-day might look like if you matriculate to this medical school, ask questions like:

- How many extracurricular activities is the typical student involved in? *Stephano, Natural Sciences major from Indiana*

- How often do you get into the city or surrounding areas? *Christian, Physics major from Oregon*

- What does a typical day look like for you? When are your exams scheduled? *Bruana, Psychology major from Connecticut*

To get a sense of what the school's environment is like:

- How close are the people in your class? Do they have a note-sharing system that people continuously use and update? How common are small co-working groups that are not mandated (e.g., Anatomy Lab groups)? *Rachael, Computer Science major from Arkansas*

- How likely are you to ask for help understanding a challenging topic? How accessible are your professors to answer questions? *Nicole, Neuroscience major from Michigan*

- Do you have an example of when faculty or school staff were particularly supportive (or not) of a student's mental health challenges? *Deeya, English major from Maryland*

To get a sense of what your future classmates might be like:

- How many students here are involved in passion projects or community service? *CJ, Speech Pathology major from Utah*

- What is the most memorable thing a student at this school has organized in the last five years? *Sarah, Public Health major from Rhode Island*

- Community service is very important to me. To what extent does the school value community engagement, and what opportunities are available to that end? *Sravya, Biology major from Massachusetts*

Asking questions not only allows you to get a feel for the school and whether or not you would fit in and be happy there, but it also has the added bonus of making you seem interested and committed to attending. In addition to the examples above, you might want to research the clubs or groups available on campus, or a dual degree program that sounds interesting. If you reach out to the admissions committee expressing interest about this before your interview, it will highlight your excitement and passion for the opportunity to learn more about the school. You'll most likely get those questions answered as well!

Remember to only ask *good* questions, though, or else your attempts will have the opposite effect. If you can google the question and find a satisfactory answer, it is the wrong question to ask in this setting. Also, if it is something super technical (e.g., what percentage of your students match into orthopedics programs?), it may be something that your interviewer or current student cannot answer for you and may lead to an awkward situation.

During Your Interview

Remember, the way you walk in the door is the first impression that the admissions committee (and potentially your future professors) will have of you.

Dress the Part

During your interview day, you want to look professional and put together. A dark-colored suit is a safe bet for men and women, but a dress with appropriate coverage and a nice sweater can also work for women, particularly if you are interviewing during the warmer months or in a warm geography. Remember, the interview day will be a long one that will likely include a campus walking tour, so it is critical that whatever you wear (footwear included!) is comfortable and practical. Interview day is a time to dress in something that makes you feel confident, classy, professional, and beautiful/handsome.

Do Not Lie

This is something that pertains to the entire application process and carries over into the interview portion. Lying or embellishing about accomplishments and time spent in an activity can be tempting, especially given the competitive nature of the application process and the fact that adcoms will rarely commit time or resources to confirming the information you have given on your activities list. Think about it: 10,000 applicants × 15 activities each? They would have to hire additional full-time staff just to go through and confirm everything that everyone writes. Highly unlikely. However, that doesn't mean that they *never* check. Statistically improbable does NOT mean impossible, and there is nothing worse for your chances of matriculation than giving an adcom even an inkling of doubt about your character and moral integrity. After all, no one wants a slimy doctor. So don't lie.

Fine, easy enough, I know, and hopefully intuitive enough advice that I wouldn't even have to write about it. However, I am including it for those of you who are even slightly, a little bit, kind of thinking about maybe, just maybe, embellishing your application *just a little bit* so that you sound more interesting. Honestly, I wouldn't have even thought it was that big a deal if I hadn't met Marcy.

At one of my first interviews, a bunch of us applicants were sitting in a room with the Associate Dean of Admissions (we'll call her AD) as we waited for our interviewers to call us in. AD had stood out to me from all of my interviews— she knew everyone one of us by name the minute we walked in the door and had clearly spent a lot of time reading through our applications. I think it was about six of us and AD in the room, having a lovely chat about the city where the school was located and what wonderful outdoor activities are available in the summer months. AD turns to a girl (let's call her Marcy) and said, "Oh Marcy, you would absolutely love it here in the summer! You could probably keep up your sailing all through medical school if you wanted to!" Marcy chuckled nonchalantly and responded something like "Oh, that sounds great," totally unscathed.

Out of nowhere, this guy, let's call him Hugh, chimes in: "Oh no way! You sail?? So does my sister! What kind of sails do you use?"

Marcy's face went B L A N K. "Uh, all different kinds. It depends on the day and weather," she responded.

Now I know that reading this, you can't actually see Marcy's face, but it is clear at this point sitting next to her that not only does Marcy not sail, but she also does not even know that sails come in different types.

Did I mention that earlier in the morning Hugh and Marcy had established that they were both from the same state? Small world. Hugh was relentlessly intrigued. "Where did you sail?" he asked.

It was too late for Marcy to back out of his, and Hugh was not getting the hint.

"Uh, on the water," she said.

I practically wanted to shake her! My mind was racing to help this girl as I tried to think of a subtle way to change the subject, but there was no in. It was like watching a train wreck you can't quite avert your eyes from.

Hugh finally figured out that this girl was probably lying and was slightly (justifiably) annoyed about it. Marcy's face went ghost white, AD gave her a very brief but judgmental side eye (mind you, AD has to stay friendly but fairly neutral throughout the entire day), and mercifully, an interviewer came to call in the next person on his roster and break the tension in what were easily the most uncomfortable 15 seconds of my young life (and yes, I was a mere observer—imagine what it was like for Marcy!).

Of course, I was not in Marcy's interview, but I can imagine that it didn't go *that* well, considering she had just gotten *destroyed* and outed in a blatant lie in front of the Dean of Admissions at this medical school. Here we have a horrific string of unfortunate, but highly unlikely, events that cost Marcy her interview and her seat at a fine medical school.

We can try to feel for Marcy here. Several students will use one of the spaces on their activities list to add a hobby that will help it stand out from the crowd. During your committee meeting someone will be able to say, "Oh, I remember her! She's that girl who sails," which is more of a distinguishable trait than, "Oh, that's that girl that volunteers." Obviously, there is some merit to this—I mean, it stood out enough to AD for her to make a comment. Points to Marcy for creativity! But learn from her mistakes. Actually *doing* interesting things is going to be much better for you in the long run than lying about it, even if it means budgeting in a gap year to your application cycle to fill it with a cool thing.

LET THEM KNOW WHY YOU WANT TO SAY YES

Let them know what you already like about their school. Admissions committees want, for practical and financial reasons, to accept people who are likely to say yes to their offer of admissions. After all, the spot they are giving you is a spot that won't be given to someone else, and if you choose not to attend, they will not only have lost a great candidate in you, but also in the other students who may commit to attendance elsewhere. There has to be some reason that you applied to this school. Was it their curriculum, philosophy, value system, or the fact that they introduce you to test patients earlier than most other schools? What about that school gets you excited about receiving your education there, and how does the design of their medical school experience fit with the way you learn and thrive? Whatever it is, tell them!

AFTER YOUR INTERVIEW

Immediately upon leaving the campus, you want to make some notes to yourself about:

- How you felt there
- What you liked/disliked
- Who you met and what you discussed (don't worry about misspelling names here; all of your interviewers will give you a business card before you leave their office)

SEND THANK YOU-EMAILS

No more than 48 hours after your interview, you will want to send an email to your interviewers thanking them for the time spent getting to know you. This email should include some details from the notes you took earlier to help your interviewer remember who you are (you probably interviewed with two people, but it is likely that they interviewed upwards of 10 students on your interview day alone). This email should be as professional as any other piece of documentation that you have sent to the medical school, as the interviewers are the people that will comment on your candidacy and influence decisions made about your application. Try something like:

Dear Dr. So-and-So,
Thank you so much for taking the time to speak with me in my interview at Amazing Medical School yesterday. I was grateful for the opportunity to learn about the school's integrative curriculum and the dual-degree program that you run. After speaking with you and several current students and learning about all the things that distinguish Amazing Medical School, I am confident that I would be very happy pursuing my medical education here. I am thrilled that my application is under consideration for such an opportunity.

Looking forward to working with you in the future,
Your Future Medical Student

To break that down: *"I was grateful for the opportunity to learn about the school's integrative curriculum and the Dual Degree program that you run,"* quickly alludes to the conversation that you had and reminds your interviewer who you are.

"After speaking with you and several current students and learning about all the things that distinguish Amazing Medical School," gives you space to mention all the things you learned in your interview that you liked about the school.

"I am confident that I would be very happy pursuing my medical education here…," establishes that you would likely attend, if accepted.

"…and am thrilled that my application is under consideration for such an opportunity," is a humble and concise way to end your email.

You want to keep this short and sweet (after all, your interviewers are all busy people), while still expressing your interest and excitement about the opportunity you were given to interview.

Send an Update Letter

Schools will each have their own policies regarding whether they accept update letters to your application. While it is worth looking into the specific policies of the schools in which you are interested, most will accept an update letter from people they have interviewed. These letters can be particularly useful for you if your application has been put on hold after your interview (i.e., you were neither immediately accepted nor rejected after interviewing at the school), or if you know that your school will be waiting to finish all of the interviews before they make a decision. More on this in the next chapter.

FOLLOW-UP LETTERS | 13

A follow-up, update, or continued interest letter can be a great opportunity for you to keep in touch with the admissions committee, express your excitement for the school, or highlight the reasons why you think you would be a better candidate for admission than anyone else.

Just like with anything else in this process, each school will have its own rules and conditions on whether they will accept additional communications from you. Some will accept letters only after you have interviewed with them, while others will accept them only if you haven't yet been invited to interview. Some accept supporting documents if you've been put on a waitlist, while others will *require* additional correspondence to keep you as an "active" applicant on that waitlist (although most won't say if this is your policy, so it is always a good idea to keep in touch after you've been waitlisted). Some med schools will prohibit you from uploading additional information altogether, others will place a limit on how much they will accept, and others will start accepting on Day 1 and won't place any limitations. In this fragmented landscape of medical school admissions policies, anything goes.

Assuming the schools you have applied to will welcome communications from the time you submit your primary application to the time they make a final decision on the state of your candidacy, there are some key times and circumstances in which these supporting documents will be most impactful.

Update Letter

If it is late in the application cycle (read: mid-December onward), and you have not been invited to an interview, send an update letter. An update letter is, as the name suggests, a quick highlight reel, updating an adcom on everything you have been up to in the six months since you last laid out your life for them on paper. What you're getting at with this letter is something like, "*In case the accomplishments and accolades I amassed over my entire pre-med career are not sufficient enough to make me competitive for your school, then maybe this additional thing that I've done more recently will put me over the edge.*"

Letter of Continued Interest

If there is a long time between the date of your interview and the date when your application will come to committee, send a letter of continued interest. For example, some schools process their interview invitations on a rolling schedule but won't make admissions decisions until they have interviewed all potential candidates. If you were to interview at a school like this in September or October and know that they won't be discussing your application in committee until February, it might make sense to send them a little nudge to remind them that you are interested in and passionate about attending.

If your application has been placed on a hold- or waitlist, you will also want to send a letter of continued interest. It is an opportunity to reaffirm your commitment to attend that school if accepted and to highlight that this is your first choice or dream school, if that is the case. In fact, some schools will factor in your demonstrated interest in the school when they are building an ordered waitlist. In that case, failing to send a letter reaffirming your interest in the school will place you at a distinct disadvantage. Similarly, depending on the month in which you will be considered for acceptance off of the waitlist, schools will have access to the gamut of results of your application cycle, complete with who accepted you, who rejected you, and what other waitlists you are on! If you have already been accepted to one school and fail to follow up with another school that has put you on a waitlist, then that school may assume that you are committed to attending the accepting school and may deprioritize you for acceptance.

What is the potential added value of spending days writing, rewriting, and editing essays that may not even be read by your admissions committee?

- It will help you to stand out, which, in a sea of qualified applicants all scrambling for a limited number of acceptance letters, is no small thing.

- It allows you to highlight your interest in the school. Your primary application will be sent to all schools, so you can't speak about any individual school at all, and several secondary applications may not give you the option of praising the attributes that have led you to apply to their school. An update or continued interest letter is an opportunity to do that.

- It grants you more space (and words) to add another dimension to your persona. You won't be able to package your entire self into roughly 10,000 words and send it to each school. However, each opportunity to share more about yourself will allow you to grow your application self into your real-life, amazing, human self and should not be taken lightly.

Hopefully I have convinced you that the potential benefits of update or continued interest letters are worth the time and effort that you will spend writing them. You should only budget about one page of space to write each, using a legible font and reasonable margins. Keep space at the top for your name, AMCAS ID number, and contact email address.

Here are some things to absolutely include in your layout.

For an Update Letter

If you are enrolled in an academic program, report your expected or final grades for the first semester. Something simple like, *"I am currently pursuing a master's degree in biomedical sciences at Fabulous University and am pleased to report I have had a strong first semester. While final grades have not yet been released, it is evident by my performance* on my midterm exams, papers, and projects thus far that my result should be a 4.0 GPA for this semester." Then you want to bring it back to them—why should they care that you did really well in this one semester of school, especially if your grades in other semesters have been less stellar? You want to anticipate all of their reservations about your application and address them in this newfound space you have available to chat with them: *"As is evident by the improvement of my grades through undergrad and now in my postgraduate work, my study habits and testing skills are continuously improving. After this additional year of work, I am confident that I will matriculate to medical school well-equipped for academic success."*

Give short descriptions of how you have spent your time since submitting your application. Draw explicit connections to how these experiences will make you a better doctor: *"Since graduating from college this past summer, I have stayed in Des Moines and continue to volunteer at the Elderly Care Home that I volunteered at as an undergrad. With more time to commit this year, I have taken on more responsibilities. I have had the opportunity to connect more meaningfully with the residents, and am proud to say that after expressing my interest in pursuing medicine, I have been entrusted with many of their medical stories. Mr. C told of the medical and nursing staff who stood in for his family in the recovery period following his heart surgery. The commitment that the staff showed and the professed impact it had on Mr. C, narrating the story so many years later, has put a face to the work and solidified my desire to become a geriatric specialist. I would be honored for the opportunity to start my journey toward serving Mr. C and others like him at your medical school."*

Finally, if you plan on making any fundamental changes to your application, such as sitting for the MCAT again or having one of your papers accepted for publication, let them know of your intentions and respectfully request that they hold off on assessing your application until those results are in. Something like this is effectively saying, *"In case you absolutely loved me but are concerned that my MCAT is too low, no worries! I'm on it, and should have a better grade to show you by the end of the month."* Something humble and simple like, *"I regret that my MCAT score is below the average for your incoming class, but I am intent on addressing that gap in my application. In fact, I have been re-preparing for the MCAT, and after making changes to my study plan, I am confident that the score, which will be released on February 11, will be competitive for your program."*

Now it is completely possible that they will ignore this request and consider your application as is, but it can't hurt to let them know that you have some good news coming up the pike.

If you are writing a letter of continued interest, you may also want to do the following:

1. Add specific details about the school that left an impression on you when you interviewed. On the interview, the school will dedicate a lot of time walking you through their buildings and associated

hospitals, and telling you about the details of their curriculum. They dedicate a lot of time and energy into "selling" their program to you over all the others. Let them know that it worked!

2. Give tidbits and information that show you have done your research. At this point in the game, you have presumably written a secondary for this school, travelled there, interviewed, and spoken with a few professors, some current students, and the Dean of Admissions. You should be able to say more about what interests you than telling them that you agree with their mission statement. Are there clubs, classes, or programs that sparked your interest? If you can see yourself spending your time volunteering in the student-run clinic on campus, let them know! If you can see yourself starting a club that you didn't see in their offerings, make a proposition. The goal here is to convince them that they would be losing out tremendously by not making you a member of their class of 20XX. Be specific, and passionate, and bold.

Sample Letters

We asked students to submit follow-up or update letters that worked for them—either by getting them an interview or by getting them off a waitlist. Here are a couple of good ones for your reference. We have blacked out any potential identifying information about the student or the receiving schools.

Sample Update Letter

"Dear ▓▓▓▓▓▓▓▓ Admissions Committee,

It is my pleasure to write to you in support of my candidacy for admission for EY 2018, and to express my continued interest in joining a cohort of ▓▓▓▓▓▓ medical students.

My interest in ▓▓▓▓ stems primarily from the fact that, in addition to providing students with a stellar medical education and clinical background, the curriculum also provides space for exploration into less traditional medical-related fields. The school's mission statement commits to improving the health of individuals and their environments in a way that is direct and comprehensive. My research and postgraduate studies in health policy and access highlight my personal commitment to this charge; seeing my passion for healthcare advocacy reflected in your curriculum is why I think I would be an excellent fit for the Class of 2022, and is why this remains among my top choice medical schools.

▓▓▓▓▓▓▓▓ is renowned for graduating committed, diligent and intelligent physicians. I believe that I can live up to the school's standard of excellence. Since graduating ▓▓▓▓▓▓ University in May, I have been pursuing opportunities to learn more about the intersection of medicine, health, and policy. [EXAMPLES HERE]

In addition to the commitment and drive that will help me to succeed academically in medical school, I am confident that the experience I will accumulate throughout this year will allow me to 'hit the ground running' next fall. I am currently [working on a research project about ▮▮. ADD EXPLANATION HERE]. I aim to submit this manuscript for publication in early 2018.

I would be honored to have the opportunity to interview at and attend the ▮▮▮▮▮▮▮. I know I could make a positive contribution to my class and to the university as a whole, and look forward to hearing from you soon. Thank you so much for your consideration."

Sample Continued Interest Letter

"Dear Mr. Dean of Admissions,

Before experiencing your school in person, my excitement to apply was grounded in tangibles: the flexible, hands-on curriculum and collaborative atmosphere are conducive to my learning style, and ▮▮▮▮▮▮▮▮, the closest 'equal access' healthcare system in the U.S. While I greatly value these components ▮▮▮▮▮▮, it was not until my interview that the intangibles that define ▮▮ emerged. The community, commitment, and inspired intellectual curiosity of the student body, as well as the administration's integration of these values into the experience have amplified my desire to join the class of 2022, and are why your school remains my top choice for medical school.

During the day I spent on campus, I expected to see students buried in textbooks—I instead joined a conversation about women's health disparities in middle-income countries, and the role of the modern physician in addressing them. I yearn to grapple with such challenging questions throughout my medical education, and would be excited to join my peers in the [CLUB NAME], who are [CLUB DESCRIPTION]. I would be excited to bring a health policy perspective to their conversation, and to guide some of the group's creative energy toward addressing the challenges in physical and financial access to care that citizens face in the surrounding city.

Secondly, I was inspired by the intellectual curiosity of the students I met, and excited at the space left in the curriculum for students to pursue the questions that drive them. Personally, my passion lies in identifying and dismantling the institutional and financial barriers that limit access to care, which I hope to explore further through a Scholarly Concentration in Health Policy. I would be excited to join ████████████████████████████ to translate my policy and medical coursework into real-world applications reforming care access. However, just by browsing through the multitude of elective offerings, research centers, and student interest groups available at ████, it is clear that each member of the class of 2022 will be approaching care delivery from a unique vantage point. Pursuing my medical education alongside classmates committed to addressing the range of issues that define "health" through the lens of their personal passions embodies my conception of what it means to be a physician of the 21st century.

It is my dream to become a physician that can address the multidimensional needs of my patients; after interviewing at ████ meeting with current students, and speaking with members of the faculty, I am confident that this is the ideal institution to make this dream a reality. I can think of no greater honor than of having the opportunity to join this community as a member of the class of 2022. Thank you again for your consideration of my candidacy to that end."

GENERAL EDITING TIPS

Finally, here are some general writing tips so that anything you send to medical schools serves to strengthen your application.

1. **Be professional. And proofread.** *A lot.* There is nothing worse for you than looking like you haphazardly slapped together this letter while trying to convince them than you want nothing more than to go to this school.

2. **Each experience should be contained within its own paragraph.** The entire document should be easily skimmable. If someone reads this, is it out of the goodness of their heart (or school policy to read everything that students submit). Either way, don't make the lives of the people you want to admit you more difficult by giving them a block of text on the page.

3. **Keep it to a page.** Because no one really wants to read more than that.

4. **Make your name, email address, and AMCAS ID clearly visible.** Again, make their lives as easy as possible—they shouldn't have to scour the text in

order to connect this piece of communication with the correct applicant.

5. **Address your reader and thank them for their time.** You are writing an ode to the medical school in the format of a letter. Be respectful to their staff.

Oh, and did I mention you should be professional and proofread? Because you should.

REAPPLYING TO MEDICAL SCHOOL | 14

We've already acknowledged (a lot) that the process of applying to medical school is a long, expensive marathon. The time between the first draft of your personal statement and the last follow-up or continued interest letter you will send can last over a year, and learning (or assuming, as some medical schools won't notify you until February or March) that you have to start all over again is going to feel like a punch in the gut. Let's get some things out in the open about this:

- It absolutely horrible to have to go through this process all over again, and you should give yourself the time and the space to acknowledge that…

- …but it is definitely NOT the end of the world, and it certainly doesn't mean that you won't get to be a doctor if that is what you want to do. All it means is that you get an extra year off before diving into your first Anatomy Lab (silver lining).

- You are not alone in facing this. According to the AAMC, of 52,777 applicants to MD-granting medical schools for admission to the Class of 2022, only 21,622 matriculated. That means that 31,155, or about 59%, of applicants last year did not matriculate.

If you have not yet received an invitation to interview by the end of November, you might begin to get anxious. By January, it is more likely than not that you are looking at bad news.

If you have received at least one invitation to interview, you will hopefully know your final status there relatively quickly. If you are accepted, celebrate! If you are rejected, think about what other interviews you have been on and how likely it seems that you will be submitting for a second application round. If you are placed on a waitlist, however, you are stuck in a sort-of limbo. You will likely have to wait until at least the end of April to hear how they will proceed with your candidacy. By April 30, applicants holding more than one acceptance will have to make a decision about which program they want to commit to, as required by the AAMC. It is at this point that schools will turn to their waitlists to begin filling open spots.

Technically, you can stay on a waitlist and still receive positive news until the first day of classes during the year for which you have applied. If an incoming student fails to show up on the first day and communicate with the school, that spot will be forfeited and the adcom will seek to fill it. Realistically, however, the chances of that happening and of you being the person they'll call are slim to none.

PLAN TO REAPPLY

When I posed the question of when applicants should plan to reapply to a former admissions counselor at a flagship state university and current admissions consultant serving over 150 students per year, she very nonchalantly responded, "As soon as you click submit the first time." I nervously giggled at this because it seemed to be about the most absurd thing I had ever heard. I remember thinking, "Uhm, maybe you haven't seen the application on our end, ma'am, but we're clicking submit for about two months by the time we finish up with all of our secondaries and then just want to breathe for a bit, not think about how likely it is for this process to fail!"

I was waiting to hear a, "Well, I'm overexaggerating a bit," but that never came.

She really did mean that you should prepare yourself to reapply as soon as you submit your application the first time around, and you shouldn't stop preparing until after you receive your first letter of acceptance—not interview, not waitlist, but actual acceptance. The good news: it is totally possible that you will receive your first acceptance letter as early as September, and that you will be able to spend almost a full year bumming around and basking in the glory of your triumph. The bad news: it is more likely that it won't be over for you so soon.

With so many stellar applicants out there, and with the average acceptance rate for MD-granting medical schools hovering at around 7% (*U.S. News and World Report*) per school for the 2017–18 school year, you have to hope for the best while bracing for the worst. The odds are just not in your favor. The challenge is that if you do have to reapply and you submit the same application again, the chances of you getting a different result than on your first attempt are slim (Am I sounding like Einstein defining insanity yet? Because that was on purpose).

Here are some things to begin mulling over sooner rather than later if you do find yourself needing to reapply.

CREDENTIALS

The number-one reason that students are not accepted to medical school the first time around is because their numbers are just not competitive enough. Look critically at the numbers that will be on your application and compare them to the averages for the schools to which you have applied using the MSAR tool. If they need to be increased, there are few ways to go about doing that:

1. If the issue is with your GPA and you are still in school, you should charge into your senior year ready to perform better than you ever have!

2. If you have already graduated from your undergraduate institution and your GPA is "closed," you may have to think about pursuing a postgraduate degree in order to get a different set of transcripts to show medical schools.

3. If the issue is with your MCAT score, study to re-take the exam while you are waiting for interview invitations and acceptance letters. Keep your content knowledge constantly refreshed, and try to weave in at least one practice passage per day into your daily

routine. It will make it much easier to take the test again if you need to.

Intangibles

Remember that medical schools are scouring your application for the values, traits, and characteristics that will make you a successful doctor and a contributing member of their incoming class. If are looking to make some changes between application cycles, these may be some good places to start.

Experiences

If you didn't do a sufficient job *showing* that you are committed to the practice of medicine the first time around, getting work as a medical scribe between application years or as you wait to receive decisions from schools can be a great way to spend your time. You will not only gain fluency in professional vocabulary that will serve you as a medical student, but the experience can also highlight your interest in the field while giving you clinical exposure in case you find yourself needing to head for Round 2.

List of schools

It may be that you are keeping yourself from gaining an acceptance to medical school because you are applying only to schools for which you are not competitive. If you are concerned that this might be the case for you, an easy fix might be to throw a few schools into the mix that report lower GPA and MCAT scores for accepted students. It may also be possible that your numbers fall short of competitive standards for MD-granting schools altogether. If that is the case, it may be worth expanding your horizons a bit further.

UNDERSTANDING DO SCHOOLS | 15

In the process of preparing this book, I spoke to hundreds of students whose credentials, activities, and qualifications for medical school ranged from the bottom decile of applicants to the top. The most common response from reapplicants to question "What would you have done differently if you could go back and alter your application cycle?" was something to the effect of *I wish I hadn't wasted time not being in medical school because I thought that DO schools were somehow inferior (or because I didn't know even know what DO schools were!)* Several of these students ended up matriculating to DO schools, and not a single one of them had originally considered these schools as viable options for them. Now in their second, third, and fourth years, they spent hours collectively on the phone with me singing the praises of these programs.

WHAT DO SCHOOLS ARE

The degree program is a DO (Doctor of Osteopathic Medicine) as opposed to an MD (Doctor of Medicine). There are 35 accredited college of osteopathic medicine across 32 states that are currently teaching 25% of all U.S. medical students. Current DO students that I spoke to likened their education to a cross between a medical degree and a physical therapist degree, and felt that the way they learned the material helped them to work confidently with their MD colleagues in patient interactions.

Differences Between MD- and DO-Granting Medical Schools

- **Application:** Applications to DO schools are centered on a different application than applications to MD schools. The AACOMAS is similar in many ways to the AMCAS application, but the personal statement to apply to DO schools, which you will submit to the AACOMAS, has a 4,500-character limit, as opposed to AMCAS's 5,300-character limit for personal statements.

- **Admissions criteria:** The average MCAT and GPA for applicants admitted to MD-granting schools in 2017/18 were 510.4 and 3.71, respectively, as opposed to a 503.1 and 3.53 for students accepted to DO schools.

- **Philosophy:** The first line of defense for treating patients for osteopaths—who prioritize healing with their hands—is different from allopaths, who turn more quickly to pharmaceutical interventions. Practically, this translates to many DO graduates tending toward primary care practice, and many MD graduates tending toward medical specialties.

SIMILARITIES BETWEEN MD-AND DO-GRANTING MD SCHOOLS

There are more similarities than differences.

- **Admissions checklist:** Applicants to both MD- and DO-granting schools must complete an undergraduate degree and all of the prerequisite courses, and must take the MCAT. They also must obtain certain extracurricular, shadowing, and clinical exposure experiences during their undergraduate and post-bac years.

- **Rights and licensure:** Both degrees confer similar rights to practice medicine—osteopaths can write the same prescriptions as allopaths and can be licensed to practice medicine in any state. Both attend four years of an accredited medical school and are taught to base diagnostic and treatment decisions on scientific evidence.

- **Professional opportunities upon graduation:** Graduates of osteopathic medical schools are able to apply to the same residency programs as graduates of allopathic medical schools, assuming they are able to take and pass the USMLE. Currently, osteopaths take the COMLEX exam, a requirement to obtain their medical license. Actually, in 2020, the two accreditation councils have plans to merge, making this a nonissue for those currently in the application process to medical school. It is true that DO graduates have lower match rates to allopathic residency programs than MD graduates, but matching to the residency of your choice is absolutely possible, regardless of which type of medical school you attend. In a report published by the *U.S. News and World Report* on the "Top 10 Medical Schools where Students Match at their First Choice Program," 50% of schools were DO granting, even though these schools make up only 19% of medical schools in the country.

WHICH ONE YOU SHOULD APPLY TO

Whether you should apply to allopathic or osteopathic medical schools will depend largely on your philosophy for the practice of medicine. However, the decision could also be made for you, depending on how well you performed in your undergraduate, post-bac, or postgraduate degrees, as well as on your MCAT. Due to the fact that the schools are newer and have, in many cases, not had the time to develop the same prestige as MD-granting schools, DO schools tend to have less competitive admissions requirements. For students who are passionate about getting a medical education but whose numbers are not competitive enough for a traditional MD program, DO schools can provide the ideal opportunity for a medical school education.

You can apply to both MD and DO schools during the same application cycle, but be aware that you will need to fill out two separate sets of primary applications. Even if the osteopathic philosophy does not thrill you and you would prefer to practice allopathic medicine, never forget that medical school is just a pit stop on the way to your career as a practicing physician. If you are able to gain acceptance to a DO school, consider it an alternative path to your career as a physician of any specialty you want. The DO education does not limit you in any way, it just opens up the field of medicine to a wider range of diverse applicants.

What to do Differently if You Want to Apply to a DO School

If you want to apply to a DO school, you should try to spend time shadowing a DO physician so that you can speak confidently and truthfully about what you like about the DO philosophy. Schools admire and prefer applicants who are applying because they are interested in osteopathic medicine, not just because they were unable to gain acceptance to an MD school. If you haven't done these things yet, speak honestly in your application about the gaps in your knowledge and work toward gaining some of that experience.

GAP YEARS AND POST-BAC PROGRAMS | 16

When I was a sophomore and junior in college, I was certain that taking a gap year between college and medical school would have ruined my life. I have immigrant parents who don't really believe in "breaks" from academics. They had all but convinced me that if I took a gap year, I would never end up going to medical school all. Even if I did go, they said, it would be about 10 times harder than if I had just gone straight through because I'd have to get myself back into the swing of studying on a daily basis.

And while the idea of being 26 years old and having just graduated from medical school seemed fine, somehow the idea of being 28 and having just graduated made me practically break out in hives. 26 years old without any money saved for a house, a car, or any real semblance of work experience (or, let's be honest, a social life) seemed fine, but 28? Twenty-eight. I could practically *feel* my roots graying and my bones getting brittle.

So when the summer after junior year came and went and I hadn't applied to medical school, I surprised even myself. I had taken my MCAT and had a competitive score (basically) and GPA for my schools of interest. So then what gives? Didn't I spend an entire chapter of this book talking about how important those two numbers are? Shouldn't that have been enough?

The problem came when I sat down to write my personal statement. As I mentioned earlier in this book, I am a pretty talkative person and write pretty quickly. So when the time came to write my personal statement outlining why I wanted to be a doctor and why I was a good candidate for medical school, I was downright cocky. I listened intently when everyone recommended that I spend a few months honing this essay and making sure each word was perfect, but in my head I was sure it wasn't going to take me more than a week to complete. When I finally did sit down to begin writing, I started to get really annoyed.

I was actually *stuck*. Why do I want to be a doctor? *Um, because that would be a cool thing to be.* Do I actually want to go to medical school? *I'm submitting the application, aren't I? You know medical school admissions people, for a bunch of doctors you don't seem to be that bright. What do you think? People take the MCAT for fun? I think that should be proof enough that I want to dedicate my life to the practice of medicine.* (To be perfectly honest with all of you, I still kind of believe that, but that is a rant for another time.)

So there I was, a junior in college, ready to apply to medical school, practically giddy with excitement as I daydreamed about all the places I would visit on my interviews and all the people I would meet in medical school and the amazing doctor I would become. So when I sat to complete one of the last outstanding things on my application checklist and realized that it just wasn't happening, you can imagine my frustration.

The process of writing the personal statement was humbling. As I tried about to write about my desire to help people through medicine, I realized that I had very little sense of what that would actually look like. "Fine," I thought. "Let's scratch this for now."

I also knew I had an interest in studying healthcare disparities and pictured myself working in underserved communities as a physician. Then I panicked. "What if I get to an interview and someone asks me why I want to that? Do I have a real answer?" I had never even shadowed in an underserved community before, and somehow "Because I want to help people" sounded incomplete, even childish. I had spent three years of college preparing myself to convince an admissions committee that I was capable of succeeding in medical school, but hadn't dedicated any time to thinking about whether or why I wanted to.

After a lot of thinking about it and second guessing myself, I ultimately decided to delay submitting my application until the end of my senior year, and essentially set myself up to take my first gap year. Despite all of my concerns, and the very real fear that I would be a grandma by the time I became a practicing physician, I ended up taking not one, but two gap years. They have turned out to be some of the most productive, fulfilling, and fun years of my life. The intuition that I had throughout the application process turned out to be not only accurate, but also a very common reason for which people might delay the application cycle. Not being *ready* to apply to medical school at the time you think you should can give you space to do many things.

Avoid Burn Out

Both pre-med and medical school can be emotionally and physically draining. Giving yourself a break for a year or two, to ensure that you are healthy and successful in the long run, is a small price to pay for a solid foundation going forward.

Set Yourself up for an Acceptance, or for the Acceptance of Your Choice

Getting med-school ready in your third year of undergrad can be quite challenging if you don't walk into college on Day 1 with your eyes set on the prize.

Similar to my experience, I have met so many students who planned on applying to medical school at the end of their junior years without putting the requisite thought into exactly what that would require. Writing a personal statement, studying for the MCAT, keeping your grades and GPA up, and saving to pay for the application while trying to maintain your sanity is quite a tall order for three short years. Unfortunately, most of this prep work can't be reasonably done much earlier than during the second semester of your junior year. For example, it is quite difficult to take the MCAT without having been exposed to all of the tested material in a classroom. While being ready to apply at this time is certainly not impossible (many people do it every year), sometimes it takes others a little bit longer to prepare all of those pieces so that they are as strong as possible, and that is completely OK, even if it doesn't feel like it at first.

Explore Other Passions or Goals

If you start medical school right after college, you will be approximately 26 years old when you graduate, after having spent eight years of your life studying. At that point, there is so much pressure to matriculate right away to a residency program, specialty, fellowship, and then official working life that it can be hard to find space to stop and catch your breath. A gap year (or two) can be an incredible opportunity to do that.

Save Up to Offset Expenses

Pretty self-explanatory. Working full time for a year can be helpful to give you a head start on some cost-of-attendances and application expenses.

Make Yourself a More Interesting Applicant

This is perhaps the most compelling reason to wait to apply to medical school, even if you are academically competitive at the end of your junior year. At the end of my sophomore year, when I began discussing application strategies with the pre-med advisor in my college's Pre-Professional Advising Office, she said something that really stuck with me: "You might be a very strong, interesting, and mature college student, but the national trend has more people waiting to apply, which means the competition gets stiffer. There is more you can do as a college graduate than you can while trying to balance everything with an academic workload." My advisor gave me an example of an alumnus at my school, Rebecca, who graduated from college, spent six months learning French and getting EMT certified, and then moved to Haiti to work on rotation in village clinics. Let me say that if I were an admissions officer trying to decide whether to admit myself or Rebecca, I would definitely pick her—and that is exactly what is happening. Rebecca and all the other Rebeccas of the world can simply speak with more evidence about their commitment to pursuing a medical degree than I can by amassing 100 hours of community service smattered across multiple semesters.

I hope I've convinced you with all of the above that it is more important to wait and apply when you're ready than it is to race for an admission when you're not. Even so, there is still the very important question of what exactly you could *do* during a gap year. Well, the world is your oyster!

After years of always being conscious of what you are doing, how well you're performing, and what that might look like to an admissions committee, you finally have a full year of time that won't be "visible" to anyone. A gap year is unique in that it will start as you submit your applications. That means there is no pressure from an admissions perspective to be impressive or productive during that time because no one will know about it anyway. There are just two important caveats to this to remember: First, you will likely be asked on many secondary applications to *briefly* describe what you plan to do during your gap year if you have already graduated from college. Second, should you find yourself on a hold or waitlist or without an interview late in the application cycle, you will likely want to send your schools an update letter. It would be pretty nice in this case if you actually had some updates to share, but thankfully, almost anything can sound interesting if you believe it is. Following are some gap year ideas, broken down by all of the motivations described above.

To avoid burn out, travel or volunteer. There are several organizations that will pay or sponsor you to teach English or volunteer abroad. As an added bonus, this cultural immersion is something interesting for you to chat about in an interview or to write about in an update letter. Just be wary of having to travel back to the United States for interviews, as that process can get expensive quite quickly.

To set yourself up for an acceptance, or for the acceptance of your choice, look critically at your application and determine which part or parts are lacking. If your grades are keeping you from applying to your chosen schools, you might want to consider getting a few more semesters of academic work under your belt through a post-bac or graduate program. If you are taking a single gap year, your senior year grades might be enough to take care of this problem. Remember that when your undergraduate GPA has "closed" after graduation, there is no altering it. Your new grades will appear in a separate GPA, but even that will have the positive benefit of demonstrating to medical schools that your grades are on an upward trend and your senior grades are at the top of that increase.

Gap years are a great way to set yourself up for success as you get more time before medical school to develop productive study habits that will serve you for life. Getting into medical school is just the start of a very long journey toward becoming a doctor. The better prepared you are going into this, the better off you will be in the long term. Similarly, if your MCAT score is the limiting factor, you can take the extra time afforded by a gap year to re-prep and re-take the exam.

If you want to take time to explore a passion or goal that was put on the backburner through your undergraduate career, a gap year is the perfect opportunity to do that! Gauri from Oregon spent her gap year in Uttarakhand, India, working and training to be a yoga instructor. Not only was this something authentic to her passions, it was interesting to discuss in her interviews and separated her from her peers. She figured that taking a year "off" from her life in the United States would not get any easier as she progressed in her medical education and career, and decided to take the leap right after graduating from college.

To save up money to offset some medical school or application expenses, a gap year can be a perfect opportunity to gain some full-time work experience. What's more, if you are able to land a job as a medical scribe, taking notes for physicians in hospitals and private practice clinics, you will be gaining fluency in medical jargon that will undoubtedly help you when you begin medical school. While it may be hard to save up enough money in a year or two to pay for the entire cost of medical school, even a small cushion to offset costs will certainly be something Future You will thank Gap Year You for. If you do manage to save enough in a couple of years to put yourself totally through medical school, please hit me up—I love to meet impressive people, and that is nothing short of impressive!

> **To become a more interesting applicant**, do things that are interesting to you and that you can write and speak compellingly about! It is really that simple.

While the idea of spending a year sitting around on an exotic beach somewhere or wasting away playing video games might sound enticing as a break between the intense years of being a pre-med and being a medical student, don't forget that a gap year will not be all fun and games. You will have to submit your primary and secondary applications, travel to interviews, and follow up with your schools, particularly as interview season draws to a close. If you do want a year that is really "off," I recommend communicating with a school that has accepted you and asking them to defer your application for a year. If you can convince them in writing that the way you will spend your time will ultimately help you to become a better doctor, more often than not they will grant your request. You do, of course, have to be prepared to hear "no," as with any request, but it is a nice way to enjoy a year away from school without the stress of the application process hanging over your head.

A final reason to pursue a gap year or two is if you plan to complete a post-bac degree in the process. This will pertain to you if you decided late in your college career, or even after completing college, that you wanted to go to medical school and/or if you did not complete the necessary pre-requisite courses while in college. There are 229 such programs registered with the AAMC today, aimed at offering continuous education programs for students who intend to pursue a medical degree but did not complete the necessary course offerings in undergrad.

Several students we spoke to reported feeling overwhelmed both by the pre-med requirements and by all the students who had been plugging away at them since first arriving on their undergraduate campuses. Post-bac programs were often brought up as suggestions for how students eased their anxiety around the application process, and then gave themselves the time to be successful in really demanding courses.

Daniel, from Virginia, started his post-bac journey while studying for a B.S. in Psychology. Originally intent on matriculating to law school and pursuing that track until the end of his junior year in college, Daniel was on the Ethics Board at his undergraduate institution. He was responsible for making judgments on appropriate punishments for students who were "brought to trial" for misdemeanors, such as cheating or financially defrauding the university. Through this activity, he found himself less interested in the judgment process and more with understanding what had compelled this student to commit this crime. He dropped his Psychology and the Law elective for Abnormal Psychology instead. In his application for a post-bac program, where he would complete the academic requirements necessary to apply to medical school, Daniel explained the impact that this switch had on his future career goals: "Abnormal Psych helped me understand the complexity and consequences of different anxiety disorders, how emotional or familial stress can affect relationships, and ultimately how people may be inclined to act in ways that deviate from their normal behavior in extenuating circumstances."

Jillian, from Connecticut who studied Nursing, followed quite a different path to her post-bac program. After being employed as a nurse for almost a decade, she was compelled to do more for her patients and to be more involved in their care. "The environment where I worked was great, but no matter how supportive your hospital is to nurses, there will always be a distinction between nurses and doctors. I found myself frustrated at carrying out orders that I had had no part in determining and thought that going to medical school could help me serve patients in a different way."

Louisa had always wanted to live abroad and applied to colleges in the United Kingdom during high school. She majored in Biology at a university in Scotland, then decided after graduation that she wanted to return to the United States to go to medical school. Louisa was frustrated to find that almost none of her schools would accept her foreign university credits toward her matriculation requirements. "The fact that I had done these requirements in another country really limited the number of medical schools that would accept my credits. I had to either do a post-bac at a university here the U.S., or resign myself to applying only to schools who accepted my credits. Honestly, I wasn't thrilled with either option, but thought that a temporary inconvenience now would be better than not being able to apply to the schools I like."

When approaching their post-bac school search, Daniel, Jillian, and Louisa each had different priorities and timelines. Daniel searched for a program that would allow him to walk through each of the pre-med courses and to engage with the material meaningfully, as if he were an undergraduate student again. He delved into a variety of offerings, "from Biology 101 all the way up to some interesting but unnecessary upper-level elective courses," and was grateful to be at a program that allowed him that flexibility. On the other hand, Jillian, who has a husband and toddler, put a premium on being able to stay close to home and to complete some courses online. She completed her post-bac education as a part-time student over three years, and was able to stay employed as a nurse and balance her busy home life in the meantime. Finally, Louisa was interested in making her understanding of the material "official" by medical school standards, and looking for a way to do so as quickly as possible. She was already confident in her knowledge of the material and just needed to make everything official through this additional year of schooling at an accredited U.S. university.

When I asked them to speak about their experiences as post-bac students, each spoke of the commitment to the program and how different it was to be engaged in a classroom full of students who were very intent on their education. Jillian noted, "I wasn't expecting to see as many people like me, with lives and kids and jobs, going back to school to do something like this. In that sense, it was much different than being an undergrad—there was no walking to a bar after class or group study sessions to make the process more enjoyable. It was really hard making time just to be there and get the material, and you could really feel that everyone was feeling the stress. At the same time, it was really amazing to be in a class where everyone is laser focused about why they're there and what they want. I feel like I learned much more than I thought I would much faster than I thought possible, and I think it was because my classmates didn't allow any space for wiggle room."

When I asked Daniel what he would have done differently in his post-bac search, knowing what he knows now in his second year, he said he wished he had been more careful in selecting the school. "A lot of post-bacs have linkage programs with the medical school at that university. I didn't realize what a benefit that could be and how much stress it would have taken off this whole process. If I could go back and do it over again, I would have done a search for a list of medical schools that I would have wanted to go to, and then picked a post-bac program at one of those schools. A lot of the linkage programs make your path to acceptance pretty straightforward, and it would have been worth a little time before I started this application process to make sure I was setting myself up for success long term."

Louisa used her time as an opportunity to work on the application. "It was kind of hard since I didn't have a GPA in the format I would need to start applying, so I didn't really know what my MCAT would have to be for me to apply to the schools I wanted. That was really a driver for me to say, "let me just aim for a 528." Setting that goal for myself really put my education into perspective. I learned the material much better than I had the first time around because I was going through my classes with an eye for preparing for the MCAT, rather than just for the midterm next month. Just changing my mindset helped everything click so much better and made me much more focused as I went through the classes. And while I didn't hit my goal score, I have to say, I was pretty darn close! Even though I was annoyed at first about having to do it, my post-bac ended up opening a lot of doors for me at medical schools that I would be really excited to attend!"

Post-bac programs serve the purpose of making medical school an option for people at all stages of their lives. Yes, it may require an extra year or two of schooling, but becoming a doctor is within the realm of possibilities for all people at any time! It just highlights the fact that if you do want to go down this road professionally, you will manage to get there somehow, and that a few years are not only small bumps in the road, but also fantastic opportunities for personal growth and development that can help make you an even better doctor.

If you have additional questions, comments or concerns as you go through this application process, or if you would like more dedicated and personalized support, please reach out directly to the author at elisabeth@makingpremedcount.com.